TRANSITION FROM SCHOOL TO YOUNG ADULTHOOD

PRO-ED Series on Transition

Edited by
J. Patton
G. Blalock
C. Dowdy
T. E. C. Smith

TRANSITION FROM SCHOOL TO YOUNG ADULTHOOD

Basic Concepts and Recommended Practices

James R. Patton
and
Caroline Dunn

pro·ed
An International Publisher
8700 Shoal Creek Boulevard
Austin, Texas 78757-6897
800/897-3202 Fax 800/397-7633
Order online at http://www.proedinc.com

pro·ed
An International Publisher

8700 Shoal Creek Boulevard
Austin, Texas 78757-6897
800/897-3202 Fax 800/397-7633
Order online at http://www.proedinc.com

Library of Congress Cataloging-in-Publication Data

Patton, James R.
Transition from school to young adulthood : basic concepts and recommended practices / James R. Patton, Caroline Dunn.
p. cm.— (PRO-ED series on transition)
Includes bibliographical references (pp. 67–70) and index.
ISBN 0-89079-782-X (alk. paper)
1. Handicapped youth—Education—United States. 2. Handicapped youth—Services for—United States. 3. Career education—United States. 4. School-to-work transition—United States. I. Dunn, Caroline. II. Title. III. Series.
LC4031.P38 1998
371.9'0473—dc21
97-47752
CIP

This book is designed in New Century Schoolbook and Melior.

Printed in the United States of America

7 8 9 10 11 12 13 14 15 09 08 07 06 05

To Kimi, that your trails be happy
and your transitions be smooth
To Tom, to the transitions ahead

Contents

Preface to Series

The transition of students from school to adulthood roles has emerged as one of the most important topics in the field of special education and rehabilitation. The critical nature of planning for the transition needs of students has also been recognized in the school-to-work, often referred to as school-to-careers, initiative.

The PRO-ED Series on Transition evolved from a symposium convened in September 1994. Along with the opportunity for professionals interested in the practical aspects of the transition process to discuss many different issues, the symposium produced a series of papers that were published originally in the *Journal of Learning Disabilities* and subsequently in bound form as a book titled *Transition and Students with Learning Disabilities.* The current series represents an attempt to provide practical resources to transition personnel on a variety of topics that are critical to the process of preparing individuals for adulthood. Each book in the series contains valuable practical information on a specific transition topic. Titles in the series include:

- *Assessment for Transitions Planning*
- *Developing Transitions Plans*
- *Follow-Up Studies: A Practitioner's Handbook*
- *Self-Determination Strategies*
- *Teaching Occupational Social Skills*
- *Transition from School to Young Adulthood: Basic Concepts and Recommended Practices*
- *Transition to Employment*
- *Working with Students with Disabilities in Vocational–Technical Settings*

We hope that these resources will add to the growing body of materials designed to assist professionals involved in the transition process. The books in this series address the need for practical resources on transition that focus solely on specific topics.

Jim Patton, Ginger Blalock, Carol Dowdy, Tom Smith

Preface

This book, which evolved out of our work in the transition area, closely represents how we convey to audiences the big picture of what transition means. Although many topics related to transition are introduced, these topics are not covered in the depth needed to affect good practice. Other books in this series accomplish this task.

This book is an overview resource that should be helpful to practitioners who need to get the overall picture of what should be done to meet the transitional needs of students. This book could be used in personnel preparation programs when the topic of transition is covered. Many programs now have coursework on transition, or at least address the topic within the structure of other existing courses. The type of information contained in this book is regularly addressed in such courses. Both of us teach courses in transition, and this book reflects how parts of these courses are taught.

We feel that the topic of transition is extremely important, as underscored by the 1990 and 1997 Individuals with Disabilities Education Act legislation. Our primary belief is that individuals experience many transitions throughout their lives and that the basic principles presented in this book hold for all of these transitions.

We also believe that the transition process involves a complex set of activities. The more proactive practitioners are in regard to preparing students for the demands of adulthood (i.e., starting early), the better off both school-based personnel and students, the primary beneficiaries, will be. As the operating guidelines presented in Chapter 1 point out, practitioners must be cognizant of key features of this process and vigilant that transition-related guidelines are instituted and maintained.

The development of any book, material, or test involves much time and energy, not all of which is provided by the authors. We recognize that many people have influenced, directly or indirectly, the final product. One of the most important people whom we want to acknowledge is Bob Stodden. Without his involvement in establishing the Hawaii Transition Project (HTP) and his desire to involve others with interests in transition, it is doubtful whether this book would be in print. His creative thinking and ongoing support of folks who worked on the HTP fostered the development of many subsequent projects, which have had a significant impact on the field. We want to acknowledge others associated with the HTP, including Phyllis Meighen Browder and Rosalie Boone, for their contributions to our thinking.

Others professionals have influenced the content contained in this book as well. Gary Clark, Mary Cronin, Ed Polloway, Lee Wiederholt, and Philip Browning have had major impacts on how we conceptualize the transition process. The editors of this series, Ginger Blalock, Carol Dowdy, and Tom E. C. Smith, have been very supportive and helpful during the development of this process.

We want to thank Alan Grimes and his production department at PRO-ED for their wonderful assistance with this project. We are particularly grateful to Chris Anne Worsham, for her help in preparing the manuscript for production and seeing that all was in order, and to Thomas Barkley, for his design of the cover. We are aware that this book would not be in print without the assistance of Chris Olson (managing editor) and Karen Swain (production coordinator), both of whom are always so nice to work with. As all authors should be, we are appreciative of the copyediting skills of Debra Berman. As always, there are people we should be naming and have failed to acknowledge. To them, we apologize but want them to know that we are thankful for their efforts.

CHAPTER 1

Basic Concepts

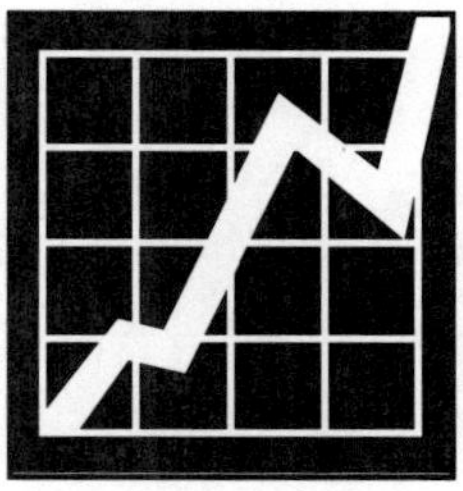

The formal study of students' transitions from school to life after high school has become popular in recent years, and the number of publications on this topic has grown significantly. The purpose of this volume is to provide a sense of the basic concepts and recommended practices associated with this process.

The notion of transition implies movement from one situation to another. Critical and not-so-critical transitions are part of everyday life for all individuals, as explained in the next section. Specific transition planning activities are mandated for only two of the many possible transitions through which children and youth with disabilities pass. First, a transition plan must be part of the Individual Family Service Plan (IFSP) for every infant and toddler eligible for services under provisions of the Individuals with Disabilities Education Act (IDEA). This plan serves to smooth the movement of these young children from early intervention to early childhood special education or another subsequent setting. Second, transition planning must be initiated by age 14 for all youth who receive special and related services under IDEA. The details of this requirement are explored in Chapter 2.

The primary focus of this book is on the transition of youth from school to postschool environments. Nevertheless, certain features affect all transitions and awareness of these features is useful to a variety of personnel.

KEY FEATURES OF TRANSITIONS

Transition typically involves change. Change is associated with new behaviors that are demanded by the new settings in which one finds oneself. It is extremely likely that, upon exit from school, young adults with special needs will experience a great deal of change as they assume new roles. This section presents a model for examining the scope and sequence of the many transitions that individuals make in their lives. In addition, this section highlights the critical elements that contribute to successful transitions.

Vertical and Horizontal Transitions

As mentioned, important transitions occur along and across everyone's life span. Some of these are normative and predictable (vertical), whereas others are individual-specific and occur at some specific point in time (horizontal). Figure 1.1 depicts the vertical transitions that individuals with disabilities will predictably experience along with select horizontal transitions that they may encounter during their lives.

The life-span–related (i.e., vertical) transitions are associated with predictable life events, such as beginning school, leaving elementary school, and

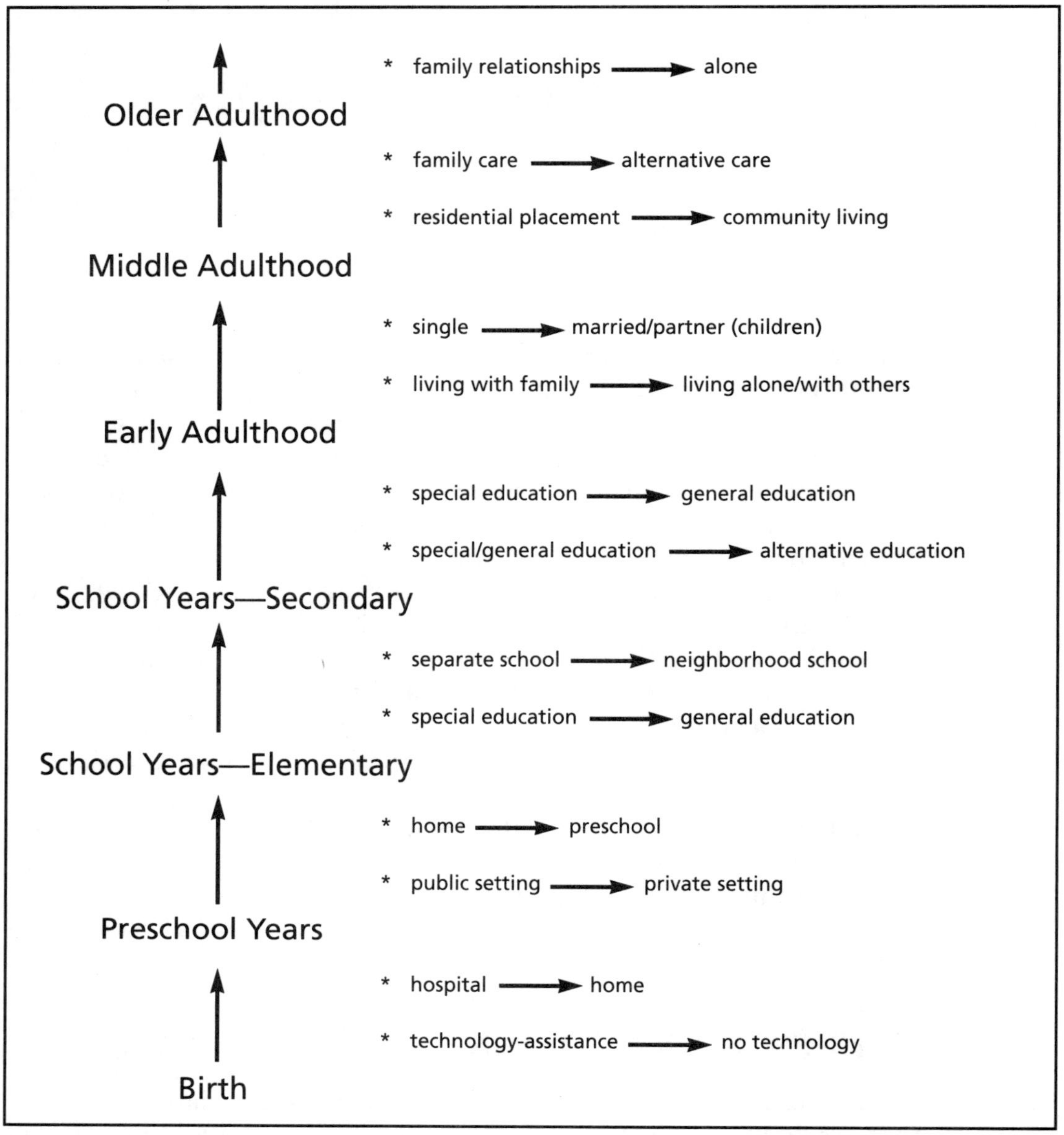

FIGURE 1.1. Vertical and select horizontal transitions. Adapted from "Transition and Students with Learning Disabilities: Creating Sound Futures," by G. Blalock and J. R. Patton, 1996, *Journal of Learning Disabilities, 29*(1), p. 8. Copyright 1996 by PRO-ED, Inc. Adapted with permission.

growing older. Coordinated planning for these transitions can minimize the anxiety that may arise, and make such transitions smoother, but in reality, little comprehensive planning occurs in the lives of most individuals.

Horizontal transitions refer to movement from one situation or setting to another. One of the most important and frequently discussed horizontal transitions is the movement from separate settings to more inclusive ones. This is an example of a transition that is not age specific, as opportunities for such movement are available throughout the life span for persons with disabilities.

Key Elements of Successful Transitions

A few key provisions allow individuals to navigate the many transitions faced throughout life. In our opinion, all transitions can be accomplished more smoothly, with reduced hassles and complications, if the following elements are in place: comprehensive planning, implementation of a plan of action, and coordination (see Figure 1.2). Although other factors, such as motivation or disposition of the person making the transition, also should be recognized as important, the basic elements highlighted in Figure 1.2 are the *sine qua non* for successful transition.

Comprehensive planning, as the figure illustrates, includes two sequential components. First, a thorough needs assessment should be undertaken. This includes examining the individual, or family, who will be going through a transition, as well as closely looking at the receiving setting into which the individual will be going. In other words, the more the professional knows about the receiving environment (i.e., what is demanded to be successful) and the existing competencies of the person who must deal with this subsequent setting, the better the chances for creating an effective transition to this new setting.

The second component, individual planning, implies that a plan of action is developed, based on an accurate needs assessment. Although this plan may be formalized in a written document, for most of the transitions listed in Figure 1.1, a document is not generated. Regardless of format, the key issue is that a plan of action is developed in which the individual's current values, personal interests, and future preferences are balanced with the realistic demands of the new settings.

Wonderful needs assessment and individualized planning are moot if the plan of action is not implemented effectively. Far too often, good plans are not put into effect. Whether the transition involves the movement of an infant with severe disabilities from the hospital to the home or the movement of an adolescent from a correctional facility back to the public school, certain actions must be accomplished to achieve the desired results. This important stage of the transition process suffers from two potential threats: (1) not being executed as planned and (2) some important aspects not being done because the needs assessment and/or the planning phase were performed inadequately.

The last key element of a successful transition is the coordination of the various parties involved in the transition itself. Such coordination requires ongoing communication and collaboration, which contribute to cooperative efforts. For example, the successful movement into an inclusive classroom setting of a student with special needs, who has never received instruction in a general education

- ***Comprehensive Planning***
  - (1) Needs assessment
  - (2) Individual planning
- ***Implementation of a Plan of Action***
- ***Coordination***

FIGURE 1.2. Key elements of successful transitions.

classroom, requires coordinated efforts between the general education and the special education staffs. Likewise, the movement of a student from school into any number of postschool settings is facilitated by coordination among various school and adult service providers.

Without comprehensive planning, effective implementation of the plan, and coordination of efforts, movement from one setting to another is likely to result only in physical relocation without the more meaningful outcomes associated with successful transition. The remainder of this book focuses on the important transition that students make from school to life after high school.

SUCCESSFUL ADULT FUNCTIONING

To understand the importance of good transition planning, it is useful to consider the outcomes associated with successful functioning in adulthood, which is the ultimate goal of transition planning efforts. Figure 1.3 depicts a simple conceptualization of the adulthood implications of transition. A brief explanation of the model, starting at the far right, follows.

In this model the ultimate outcome for which all transition efforts should be directed is to help create lives that are characterized by personal fulfillment. This concept relates closely to the notion of quality of life, as discussed by Halpern (1993). Halpern suggested that quality of life—or personal fulfillment—relates to three elements: happiness (transient state of affect), satisfaction (feelings and behavior patterns associated with different adult roles), and sense of general well-being (enduring sense of satisfaction with one's life). We believe that all that professionals do with students should be guided by the overriding theme of enhancing the students' quality of life by imparting the means for them to be personally fulfilled.

To enjoy some sense of personal fulfillment, an individual must be reasonably successful in meeting the challenges of everyday life, whether at work, at home, in school, or in the community. Various references (Brolin, 1993; Cronin & Patton, 1993) provide listings of the major demands encountered in adulthood. People who feel that they are personally fulfilled do not always deal successfully with the day-to-day issues that arise in their lives; however, they are more likely than other individuals to handle those issues successfully most of the time.

How does one become competent to deal with the daily challenges of life? Three factors are essential. First, an individual must have knowledge of an array of facts, procedures, and events that are part of his or her postschool environments. Second, the individual needs to acquire specific skills typically demanded in the assortment of settings in which the person must function. Third, the person must identify, access, and use a host of supports and/or services that will be of great assistance in dealing with everyday events.

It is possible to think of the individual supports and services as related (see Figure 1.4). Although Luckasson and colleagues (1992) suggested that services are "a subset of supports or . . . a type of support" (p. 144), a slight distinction is used in this book as follows: *Supports* involve a variety of resources, including other people (e.g., family, friends, co-workers) or technology (e.g., assistive devices), whereas *services* are either generic (i.e., available to all in the community such as community mental health services) or specialized (i.e., services, such as vocational rehabilitation or personal care attendants, for which one usually has to be determined eligible under some set of criteria). The interesting point is that everybody uses supports and services throughout life and the idea of seeking such support is a natural part of life.

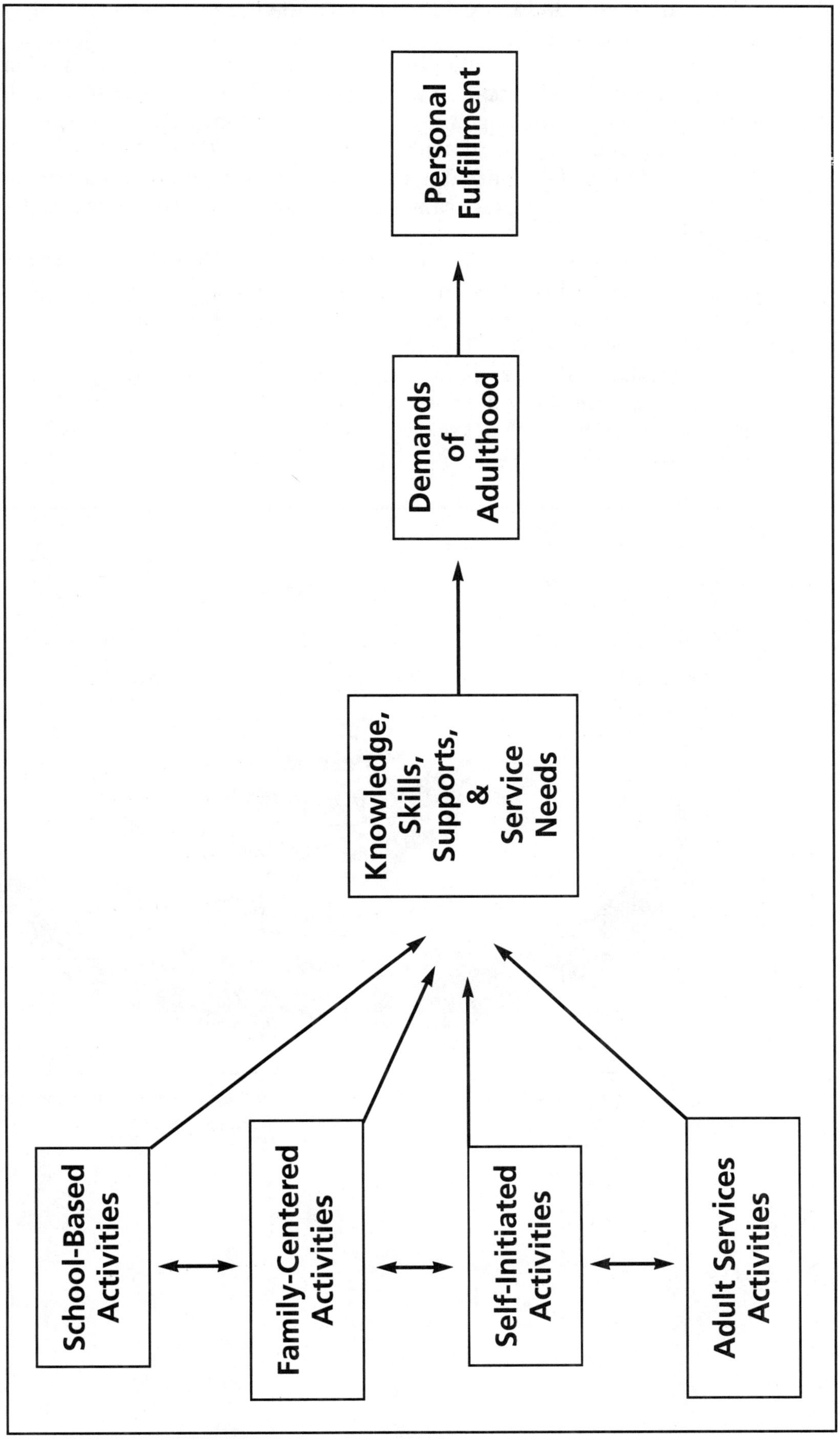

FIGURE 1.3. Adulthood implications of the transition process.

As can be seen in Figure 1.3, four entities share the responsibility for preparing students for adulthood. These four elements—school, family, the student, and adult services—are intricately involved in the transition process. Ideally, efforts to prepare students for dealing with the everyday issues of adulthood begin early in school as part of the ongoing education of students. This proactive approach to transition can be considered transition education (Clark & Kolstoe, 1995). Transition efforts that begin around age 14 are more reactive in nature and are limited to a more narrow time frame (i.e., the amount of time a student remains in school).

It is important to recognize that the process whereby students are taught the knowledge and skills, as well as linked to the supports and services, that they will need later on is a shared responsibility. Whereas the school operates under the mandate of the transition planning process and should take the lead in this effort, the family, the student, and other service providers also play critical roles. In reality, however, these other players might not contribute substantially to the overall process. When this is the case, school-based personnel will likely need to play a larger role.

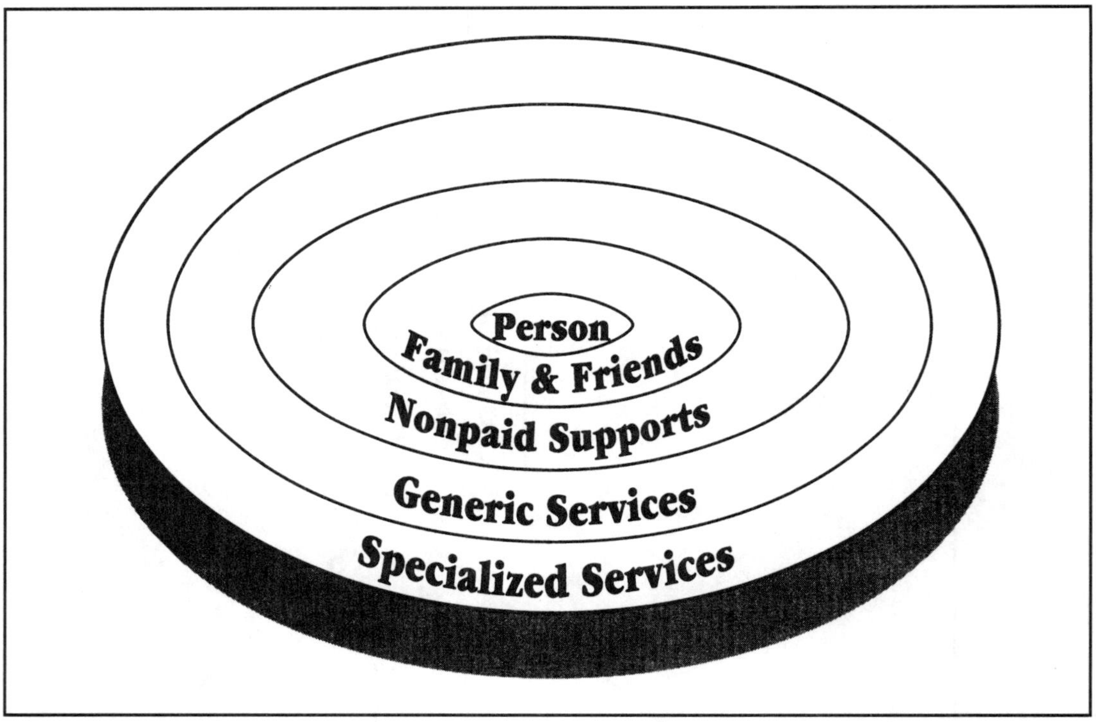

FIGURE 1.4. The nature of systems of supports. From *Mental Retardation: Definition, Classification, and Systems of Supports* (9th ed., p. 144), by R. Luckasson et al., 1992, Washington, DC: American Association on Mental Retardation.

CHAPTER 2

Nature and Background of the Transition Process

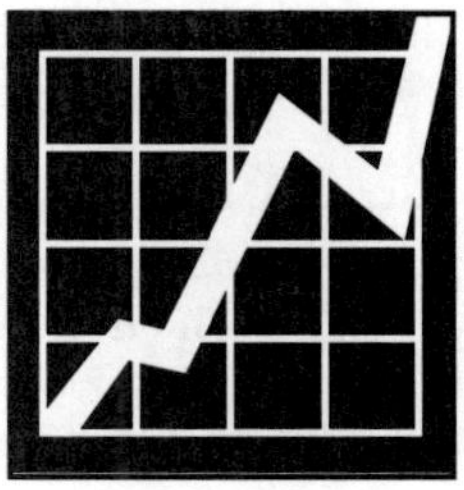

RATIONALE FOR TRANSITION PLANNING

In addition to the obvious reasons why transition planning is a good idea, as cited in the previous chapter, other reasons exist for implementing such efforts, as supported by research findings. Three factors, each of which provides a strong rationale for recommending that comprehensive transition planning be conducted, are discussed in this section.

Adult Outcome Data

One of the most significant factors that added support to the beginning of the transition movement was the data on the adult outcomes of students who had been in special education for substantial periods of their school careers. Research results substantiated a rather bleak picture of unemployment—long-term underemployment for those individuals with jobs; minimal participation in postsecondary education, with even bleaker completion rates; few individuals living independent lives; limited social lives; and little community involvement (Hasazi, Gordon, & Roe, 1985; Mithaug, Horiuchi, & Fanning, 1985; Sitlington, Frank, & Carson, 1993; Wagner et al., 1991).

A sampling of outcomes from the National Longitudinal Transition Study (Wagner, Blackorby, Cameto, Hebbeler, & Newman, 1993) in the areas of postsecondary education, employment, residential independence, social domain, and citizenship is highlighted in Table 2.1. Although specific outcomes sometimes vary depending on the type and nature of the disability, far too often the outcomes are significantly less than what is found for students without disabilities.

Exit Data

Another area of concern is the high dropout rates for students with disabilities. Although dropping out is only one of the ways students exit school, the dropout rates of students with disabilities are disturbing (see data provided in Table 2.2). These rates are a concern because dropping out removes students from school, where they might acquire the knowledge and skills or be linked to the supports and services they undoubtedly will need. The implication of the dropout rates is that transition planning must start early to be useful for those students who will not graduate with a diploma, earn a certificate of completion, or age out.

TABLE 2.1

Outcomes from the National Longitudinal Transition Study

- *Postsecondary education.* Few students with disabilities went on to postsecondary education. When they had been out of high school 3 to 5 years, fewer than one-third had done so, less than half the rate of youth in general. College attendance was particularly low. Enrollment rates were lowest for youth with learning disabilities and mental retardation; youth with sensory impairments enrolled at rates similar to typical youth.
- *Employment.* There were strong gains in employment over time, so that 57% of youth with disabilities were competitively employed when they had been out of school 3 to 5 years. This rate was still lower than that for the general population of youth. Significant increases for youth with disabilities were noted in the proportion of youth working full time and in those earning more than $6 per hour. Gains were experienced largely by youth with learning, speech, or emotional disabilities; employment trends for most other disability categories were flat.
- *Residential independence.* Youth with disabilities showed a significant increase in independent living after high school; 37% lived independently 3 to 5 years after leaving school. However, this rate was substantially below the rate of youth as a whole. Independent living was more common among employed youth and those earning higher wages, as well as among females, because women were more likely to be married.
- *The social domain.* The rate at which youth belonged to groups and saw friends declined over time, although social isolation was rare; only 5% of youth saw friends less than weekly, did not belong to any community groups, and were not married or engaged. This rate was 25% for youth with multiple impairments. Overall, youth with disabilities were married or living with someone of the opposite sex when they had been out of high school 3 to 5 years at about the same rate as typical youth. However, young women with disabilities were significantly more likely than their nondisabled peers to be mothers (41%), particularly single mothers (20%).
- *Citizenship.* Half of youth with disabilities were registered to vote when they had been out of school 3 to 5 years, compared with two-thirds of youth in the general population. Registration rates were higher among high school graduates than among dropouts. Arrest rates rose sharply. Overall, 19% of youth with disabilities out of high school up to 2 years had been arrested at some time; 3 years later the rate was 30%. Arrests occurred primarily to youth with serious emotional disturbances, among whom 58% had been arrested.

Note. From *The Transition Experiences of Young People with Disabilities: A Summary of Findings from the National Longitudinal Transition Study of Special Education Students* (p. 3-1), by M. Wagner, J. Blackorby, R. Cameto, K. Hebbeler, and L. Newman, 1993, Menlo Park, CA: SRI International. Copyright 1993 by SRI International. Reprinted with permission.

Curricular Issues

A third factor that underscores the need to conduct comprehensive transition planning relates to the nature of the curriculum to which students with disabilities are exposed. The use of functionally oriented curricula has been identified by teachers as critical to improve instruction for students with disabilities at the secondary level (Halpern & Benz, 1987). The importance of functional curricula has

TABLE 2.2

Dropout Data for Three Select Groups

	Percentage of Students Who Dropped Out	
Category of Disability	**NLTS**	**DOE**[a]
Learning disabilities	29	18.8–28.5
Emotional disturbance	48	24.0–39.0
Mental retardation	30	19.0–27.0

Note. NLTS = National Longitudinal Transition Study (Wagner et al., 1993). DOE = U.S. Department of Education (1995).

[a]Indicates a potential range, with the first figure representing the listed dropout rate and the last figure representing the combination of the dropout figures plus those of the unknown exit category.

also been recognized and championed by the Division on Career Development and Transition (Clark, Field, Patton, Brolin, & Sitlington, 1994).

One way to examine how well curricular efforts are developing everyday living skills is to ask parents about the functional abilities of their sons and daughters. Wagner and colleagues (1993) surveyed parents of children from a variety of disability areas; their findings are provided in Table 2.3. In looking at the aggregate data for all conditions, it is startling to note that a substantial percentage of youth, as perceived by parents, do not demonstrate adequate functional abilities in the areas of functional mental skills (43.1%) and community living skills (38.6%). It is important to understand the distinctions among the different types of skills reported in this table, as described in the footnotes. Nevertheless, most professionals would agree that students should be taught these skills in school and demonstrate proficiency before exiting the system.

HISTORICAL PERSPECTIVE

A number of historical events have influenced the evolution of transition planning and transition activities. Current practice has been preceded by efforts that occurred primarily in the mid-1980s. These efforts were characterized by attempts to systematically examine the importance of formalizing the process to prepare students for adulthood more effectively.

In reality, transition activities have been operative for quite some time in many locations across the country. In the past, transition activities were called something else and may have overlooked certain types of students with disabilities (e.g., those with learning disabilities). For decades, certain school personnel have been assisting students in making the transition from school to community

TABLE 2.3

Functional Abilities by Disability Category

	Percentage of Youth with Parents Reporting:		
Disability Category	**High Self-Care Skills[a]**	**High Functional Mental Skills[b]**	**High Community Living Skills[c]**
All conditions	86.4	56.9	61.4
Learning disabled	95.5	66.0	74.2
Emotionally disturbed	94.1	65.3	66.9
Speech impaired	91.8	68.9	67.3
Mentally retarded	67.4	32.8	29.4
Visually impaired	51.6	31.8	41.2
Deaf	83.4	44.3	43.4
Hard of hearing	92.3	60.7	45.8
Orthopedically impaired	42.3	50.5	32.5
Other health impaired	65.3	57.3	41.2
Multiply handicapped	34.5	12.8	21.3
Deaf/blind	21.0	6.8	13.2

[a]Skills include dressing oneself, feeding oneself, and getting around outside the home. Scale ranges from 3 to 12. High is 12.

[b]Skills include counting change, reading common signs, telling time on an analog clock, and looking up telephone numbers and using the phone. Scale ranges from 4 to 16. High is 15 or 16.

[c]Skills include using public transportation, buying clothes, arranging a trip out of town, and using community resources, such as a swimming pool and/or library. Scale ranges from 4 to 16. High is 15 or 16.

Note. From *The Transition Experiences of Young People with Disabilities: A Summary of Findings from the National Longitudinal Transition Study of Special Education Students* (p. 2-13), by M. Wagner, J. Blackorby, R. Cameto, K. Hebbeler, and L. Newman, 1993, Menlo Park, CA: SRI International. Copyright 1993 by SRI International. Reprinted with permission.

life. For instance, many of the work–study programs of the 1960s contained aspects of the transition process that are being espoused today. In addition, many families have done a superlative job of readying their adolescent children for the realities of adulthood.

Models of Transition

The beginning of the transition movement, as it is known today, is often associated with the initiatives that derived from the Office of Special Education and Rehabilitative Services (OSERS). Arguably, Will's (1984) document provided a sense of the federal government's policy, which envisioned transition as "an outcome-oriented process encompassing a broad array of services that lead to employment" (p. 1).

This "bridge-from-school-to-working-life" conceptualization of transition, as shown in Figure 2.1, emphasized employment as the primary outcome on which training and linkages should be based. This model identified different levels of services that might be needed to achieve desired employment outcomes and recognized that nonvocational dimensions of adulthood are important, but only as they relate to the employment goal (Halpern, 1985).

This parochial view of adult outcomes was broadened in a well-received alternative conceptualization developed by Halpern (1985). Halpern recommended that two additional dimensions—the quality of one's residential environment and the adequacy of one's social and interpersonal networks—be viewed as equally important factors contributing to successful community adjustment. Halpern's revision of the original OSERS model, as shown in Figure 2.2, reflected the emerging notion that transition must be more comprehensive.

During the mid-1980s, a number of federally funded projects began to study the transition process. As these projects began to disseminate their work, it became clear that transition services and planning involved the consideration of many different areas. Today, models of transition typically include consideration of a comprehensive list of transition areas, some of which are employment, further education and training, daily living, leisure, community participation,

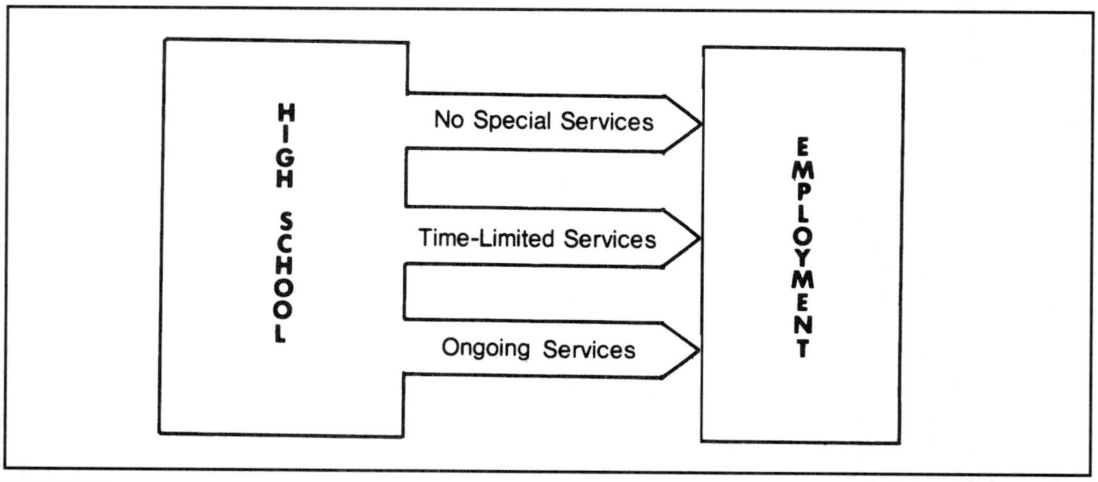

FIGURE 2.1. OSERS transition bridge model. From *OSERS Programming for the Transition of Youth with Disabilities: Bridges from School to Working Life,* by M. Will, 1984, Washington, DC: Office of Special Education and Rehabilitative Services.

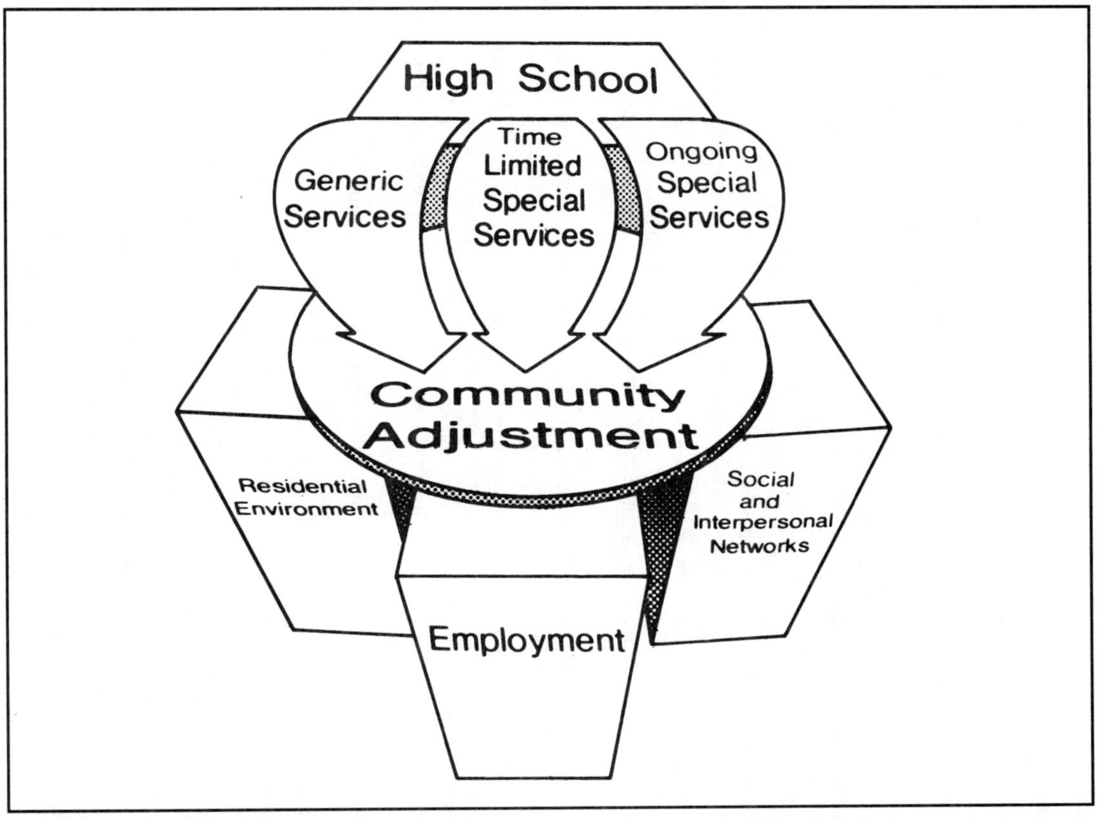

FIGURE 2.2. Halpern's transition model. From "Transition: A Look at the Foundations," by A. S. Halpern, 1985, *Exceptional Children, 51,* p. 481. Copyright 1985 by The Council for Exceptional Children. Reprinted with permission.

health, relationships and social interactions, financial and money management, and transportation.

Federal Legislative Mandates

Another measure of the growing importance and changing conceptualization of transition is found in the legislation enacted over time. Many pieces of federal legislation have addressed the issue of transition; Table 2.4 lists chronologically some of the most important laws and includes a brief description of the impact these laws have had on transition efforts.

One of the most important pieces of legislation that has had a significant impact on transition is the Individuals with Disabilities Education Act of 1990 (IDEA). The 1990 amendments to the original Education for All Handicapped Children Act of 1975 are particularly noteworthy because, for the first time, transition services were mandated for all students who were eligible for special education and related services. Statements of needed services must be in place by age 16. Prior to 1990, many states provided various degrees of transition services; however, IDEA mandated that all states had to comply with federal regulations. In 1997, IDEA was reauthorized and additional changes, as noted in Table 2.4, were instituted. One of the most important changes is that the transition process now must commence at an earlier age, with a statement of transition needs being developed prior to age 14.

(text continues on page 14)

TABLE 2.4
Select Federal Legislation Related to Transition Services

Year	Legislation	Public Law	Transition Implications
1973	Rehabilitation Act	93-112	Section 503 requires employers receiving federal contracts to take affirmative action to recruit, hire, train, and promote individuals with disabilities. Section 504 is considered the first civil rights law protecting the rights of individuals with disabilities. Section 504 statute reads, "No otherwise qualified handicapped individual in the United States shall, solely by reason of his handicap, be excluded from participation in, be denied the benefits of, or be subjected to discrimination under any program or activity receiving Federal financial assistance."
1975	Education for All Handicapped Children Act	94-142	Mandated free, appropriate public education for all children and youth with disabilities, including special education and related services. A written Individualized Education Program (IEP) must be developed and implemented for all children and youth eligible for special education or related services.
1976	Vocational Education Act Amendments	94-482	Extended the provision of vocational education services to individuals with disabilities of all ages. Secondary and postsecondary programs receive funds, of which a percentage must be spent on special populations. Vocational education plans for youth with disabilities must be coordinated with the youth's IEP.
1978	Rehabilitation, Comprehensive Services, and Developmental Disabilities Act Amendments	95-602	In 1981, this law was interpreted by the Rehabilitation Services Administration to allow persons with severe learning disabilities to receive rehabilitation services.
1982	Job Training Partnership Act (JTPA)	97-300	Established programs to prepare youth and unskilled adults for entry into the labor force and to afford job training to those economically disadvantaged persons, and other persons facing serious barriers to employment. Persons with disabilities are eligible for JTPA training. Youth with disabilities can participate in programs funded under JTPA programs while in secondary school as well as after exiting secondary school.
1983	Education of the Handicapped Act Amendments	98-199	Established a new grant authority to fund programs to improve secondary special education and transitional services for youth with disabilities (§ 626). Many programs offering transition services for youth with disabilities have been initiated using these funds.
1984 & 1986	Rehabilitation Act Amendments	98-221 98-506	Increased the emphasis on services to youth with disabilities. In the 1986 amendments to the Rehabilitation Act, the state plan requirements were changed to require states to (a) plan for individuals who are making the transition from school to work, and (b) reflect how the state rehabilitation agencies will implement the new supported employment program.
1984	Carl D. Perkins Vocational Education Act	98-524	Strengthened provisions and assurances to youth with disabilities, including access to the full range of vocational program offerings in the least restrictive environment and the provision of vocational assessment prior to students entering vocational education.
1990	Carl D. Perkins Vocational and Applied Technology Education Act	101-392	Significant funding changes were made in this legislation, but the assurances for special populations were maintained and the emphasis on transition support increased. In addition, vocational education is expected to coordinate efforts with vocational rehabilitation as well as special education. This legislation established a technical preparation program (Tech Prep) that begins with 2 years of preparation in secondary school, followed by 2 years of training in community college.

(*continues*)

TABLE 2.4. *Continued.*

Year	Legislation	Public Law	Transition Implications
1990	Individuals with Disabilities Education Act	101-476	(Formerly Education of the Handicapped Act) Defined transition services as follows (§ 602(a) 19)): a coordinated set of activities for a student, designed within an *outcome-oriented* process, which promotes movement from school to postschool activities. In § 602(a)(20) a requirement was added that IEPs include a statement of the needed transition services for students beginning no later than age 16 and annually thereafter (and, when determined appropriate for the individual, beginning at age 14 or younger), including, when appropriate, a statement of the interagency responsibilities or linkages (or both) before the student leaves the school setting.
1990	Americans with Disabilities Act	101-336	Guarantees equal opportunity for persons with disabilities in employment, public accommodations, transportation, state and local government services, and telecommunications.
1992	Rehabilitation Act Reauthorization	102-569	Directs state rehabilitation agencies to address working with youth with disabilities in the state plan. Intention is to reduce service gaps between education and rehabilitative services when these are needed for exiting students. The legislation intends to strengthen the coordination between vocational rehabilitation and the schools, including exchange of information and data, provision of services, and access to rehabilitation services.
1994	School-to-Work Opportunities Act	103-239	Promotes the development of transition programs for all students. Demonstrating cooperation at the federal level, selected funding from the U.S. Department of Education and the U.S. Department of Labor are combined to provide money to establish statewide systems for school-to-work opportunities for all students. In addition to state funds, the act also provides grants to local *partnerships* that include broad community representation, including people with disabilities.
1997	Individuals with Disabilities Education Act Reauthorization	105-17	Added related services to the coordinated set of activities offered to students with disabilities as transition services. Added the requirement that by age 14, IEP communities address transition goals, including the secondary education course offerings that facilitate achieving postschool transition goals. Clarified that all rights given to parents under IDEA transfer to students who reach the age of majority (18 in most states) and who can give informed consent. Expanded the emphasis on the inclusion of students with disabilities in statewide assessment and required that an alternate assessment be developed for students who do not participate in statewide assessment.

Note. Adapted from *Transition and School-Based Services: Interdisciplinary Perspectives for Enhancing the Transition Process,* by S. deFur and J. R. Patton (Eds.), in press, Austin, TX: PRO-ED; and "Transition of Youths with Learning Disabilities to Adulthood: The Secondary Education Foundation," by S. deFur and H. B. Reiff, 1994, in *Learning Disabilities in Adulthood: Persisting Problems and Evolving Issues* (pp. 101–102), by P. J. Gerber and H. B. Reiff (Eds.), Austin, TX: PRO-ED.

Definitions of Transition

Transition from school to postschool settings has been defined in different ways. As mentioned, Will's (1984) definition stressed that transition is "an outcome-oriented process." This fundamental idea was retained in the definition of transition services contained in IDEA (1990):

> a coordinated set of activities for a student, designed within an outcome-oriented process, which promotes movement from school to post-school activities, including post-secondary education, vocational training, integrated employment (including supported employment), continuing and adult education, adult services, independent living or community participation. (§ 602(a)19)

Because the IDEA definition of transition services remained unchanged in the 1997 reauthorization, it will continue to be used as the federal reference for defining transition.

Other definitions of transition have been developed by various sources. One of the most comprehensive definitions, reflecting the best blend of contemporary thinking on this topic, was adopted by the Division on Career Development and Transition (DCDT) in 1994. This definition underscores the realities associated with change. It points out that, as students leave school, they will have to assume a variety of adult roles in the community. It also stresses the proactive aspects of transition education and the importance of actively involving students in this process whenever possible. The definition, written by Halpern (1994), reads as follows:

> Transition refers to a change in status from behaving primarily as a student to assuming emergent adult roles in the community. These roles include employment, participating in post-secondary education, maintaining a home, becoming appropriately involved in the community, and experiencing satisfactory personal and social relationships. The process of enhancing transition involves the participation and coordination of school programs, adult agency services, and natural supports within the community. The foundations for transition should be laid during the elementary and middle school years, guided by the broad concept of career development. Transition planning should begin no later than age 14, and students should be encouraged, to the full extent of their capabilities, to assume a maximum amount of responsibility for such planning. (p. 117)

GUIDING PRINCIPLES

Certain principles are essential to guiding the transition process for students with special needs. The 13 guiding principles discussed below have been gleaned from the professional literature on transition and from actual practice. They should serve as a frame of reference for the implementation of transition services.

▶ **1. Transition efforts should start early.**

This point has already been made in this book and has been validated by other sources (DCDT definition). Without question, it is preferable to consider the transition process from a proactive rather than a reactive perspective. Certain precursors of the knowledge and skills needed in adulthood can be started at the preschool level. Most can be addressed before transition needs are assessed prior to age 14. What is needed is a systematic K through 12 transition education program that has a strong base at the elementary level (Clark, Carlson, Fisher, Cook, & D'Alonzo, 1991).

Families should be informed of the transition process early on. They can be provided information that they need to be considering as their child moves through school. Some transition-related activities must be started early to ensure a seamless transition to postschool settings.

▶ 2. Planning must be comprehensive.

This principle has already been highlighted. The main point is that a range of adult outcome areas should be evaluated when a needs assessment is conducted. If a strong proactive transition education program is in place, then fewer areas of need are likely to be identified. Nevertheless, a comprehensive look at each student must be performed and dismissal of some transition planning areas should not be done as a function of the student's disability. For instance, the transition needs of certain youth, particularly those with learning disabilities, may be overlooked because of the misconception that these students do not have needs in some areas (e.g., daily living). The data in Table 2.3 on functional abilities, however, suggests that a number of young adults with learning disabilities do need to acquire basic functional skills.

▶ 3. Planning process must balance what is ideal with what is possible.

It is easy in a book like this to recommend that transition services should be comprehensive and suggest that a great amount of effort be put into the transition process for each student. Although this recommendation is sound and the accompanying suggestions warranted, the realities of serving large numbers of students must be taken into consideration. The practices associated with sound transition planning must be acceptable to those who have to carry them out. This concept, known as *treatment acceptability,* is an important one to understand and keep in mind when developing transition services.

Recommended practices need to be immediately useful to school-based staff and cannot be time demanding. Some transition specialists have extremely large caseloads and are unable to conduct in-depth assessment of every student. Techniques and methodologies are needed that provide as much information as possible within a reasonable amount of time and with a reasonable amount of effort.

▶ 4. Student participation is essential.

The literature on transition regularly stresses the importance of preparing students to be active, contributing participants in their transition planning process. They should be because it is their lives that are being discussed and about which decisions are being made. The physical presence of students at their transition planning meeting is not sufficient; they should be the driving force behind this process and the meeting. Of course, this will not always be possible, as some students are not capable of directing their transition planning process. However, far too few students who are capable, are active contributors.

In recent years, a number of curricular materials focused on teaching students how to become active players in the planning process have become available. Two notable examples of this type of material are *Next S.T.E.P.: Student Transition and Educational Planning* (Halpern et al., 1997) and *Self-Directed IEP* (Martin, Huber Marshall, Maxson, & Jerman, 1996), which is part of the ChoiceMaker Self-Determination Curriculum.

► 5. Family involvement is crucial.

As illustrated in the model shown in Figure 1.3, families play a key role in the shared responsibility for preparing their children for dealing successfully with the challenges of life. Moreover, for most young adults with disabilities, it is their parents or guardians who become their service coordinators, or transition specialists once school ends. For these reasons, it is imperative that parents and guardians become informed, skilled, and active in the transition process. Clark and Patton (1997) suggested that, in addition to determining the preferences and interests of students, it is valuable to do likewise with families.

Transition professionals must not become disillusioned by the fact that a substantial number of parents and guardians either will choose not to assume the important role discussed above or will be ineffective in this role. During the time the student is still in school, it is possible and necessary for school-based personnel to take responsibility for certain critical activities that the families should do. After students exit from the school system, they and their families must realize that they likely will be on their own without the supports they have previously had available.

One idea that comes from the practices associated with early intervention services is to conduct transition planning activities such as those used in the development of the Individual Family Service Plan (IFSP). One of the components of the IFSP is information on the family's strengths and needs. This information is used to assist in the development of services that will benefit the infant or toddler. Similarly, it may be useful to assess a family's strengths and needs when generating transition plans, particularly when determining who is responsible for making important contacts with adult service providers.

Transition personnel must respect family values. It is important to recognize that families will base their requests, opinions, and comments on their own community or cultural values, practices, and traditions. Their perspectives must be respected, even when in conflict with those of school-based personnel.

► 6. The transition planning process must be sensitive to diversity.

There is no question that the transition process is affected by the changing demography in this country (Patton, Cronin, & Jairrels, 1997). Heightened awareness of cultural diversity has emerged in recent years. Although sensitivity to specific cultural distinctions must be instituted, cultural diversity is only one type of diversity that must be addressed. Other dimensions that should be considered are displayed in Figure 2.3. Although all of these elements are worthy of attention, some are less obvious than others. For instance, the implications of gender in the transition process may be so subtle that they are overlooked. Female students, for example, should not be limited in their consideration of vocational options; they should be afforded a wide range of choices.

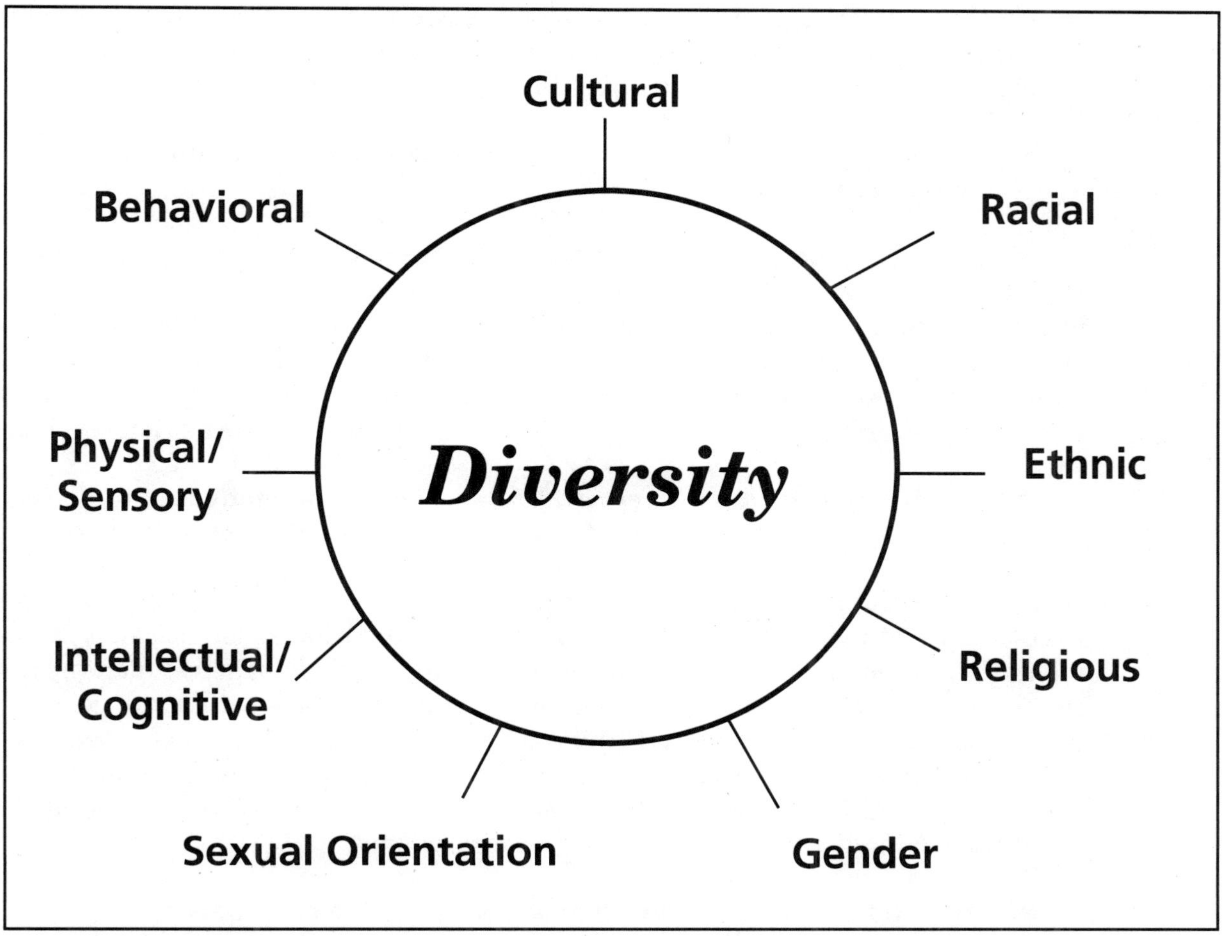

FIGURE 2.3. Diversity that must be addressed in the transition planning process.

▶ 7. Everyone uses supports and services.

We are all, as Condeluci (1995) noted, interdependent beings. It is very natural to use supports that exist in our everyday environments. We ask co-workers for rides to work when our cars are in the shop. We drop off our children at their grandparents' houses when we need to be away from home. We pay folks to cut our grass, pick up our garbage, dry clean our clothes—we use community services regularly. None of us find anything wrong with it.

With this in mind, it is essential that professionals convey to youth with special needs that the use of supports and services is acceptable and useful. These individuals need to be taught when and how to use the array of natural supports and services available to them in the settings in which they live, work, and play.

▶ 8. Community-based activities are important.

Most students with disabilities will prosper from experiences that are provided in real-life contexts. These students are more likely to acquire the knowledge and skills they will need to function in community settings if they have opportunities to learn and practice in these settings.

Community-based assessment and instruction are strongly recommended for determining one's needs and providing meaningful learning. One of the strongest reasons for delivering instruction in community settings is that many individuals with disabilities have difficulty generalizing the skills they have learned in the classroom to community settings (Dunn & Rabren, 1997).

▶ 9. Interagency commitment, cooperation, and coordination must be improved.

Adult service providers are key players in the transition process, as implied in Figure 1.3. Most adult service agencies, whether public or private, are responsible for a wide range of services, and transition is not one of their major charges. However, to enhance the overall effectiveness of the transition planning process, adult service providers must be involved. As a result, efforts must be ongoing to improve the coordination of various agencies and school-based transition services.

▶ 10. Timing is crucial if certain linkages are to be made and a seamless transition to life after high school is to be achieved.

Changes associated with the reauthorization of IDEA provide a strong message that the timing involved with the transition planning process is critical. A statement of transition needs is now required by age 14 for all identified students. This requirement improves the chances that appropriate plans will be developed, needed services will be identified, and requisite activities will be performed.

The overall goal is to move the student from school to various subsequent settings without difficulty and without the interruption of needed services. Only when the timing is right can this goal be accomplished.

▶ 11. The transition planning process should be considered a capacity-building activity.

Considering a student's transition needs is by definition a deficit-oriented process. Although deficits cannot be totally ignored, this process should promote the recognition of the student's strengths as well. A thorough needs assessment should determine both areas of concern and areas in which the individual shows competence and proficiency. Transition staff need to consider both aspects of the student's profile.

▶ 12. Ranking of transition needs must occur.

Some youth will display an extensive list of needs. It is important not only to identify these needs, but also to determine which ones should be addressed first. If the student is likely to exit school in the near future, a ranking of needs must be done. This ranking can be based on a number of factors, such as which areas are most critical for successful adult functioning or which areas the individual will encounter first. The priority ranking should be determined by the student when appropriate.

▶ 13. Transition planning is beneficial to all students.

When one thinks about the concept of transition planning, it does not take long to realize that it is a good idea for *all* students. Most students in fact leave school underprepared for young adulthood. Even those students who go to the most respected schools, who grew up in loving and nurturing families, and who are intelligent in their own right, are very likely to go to college or enter the workforce without the knowledge and skills to deal successfully with the demands of everyday life.

To date, systematic transition planning is required only for students who are eligible for services under IDEA. However, rumblings are beginning to be heard in other quarters. The National Association of Secondary School Principals (NASSP) (1996), in their document titled *Breaking Ranks: Changing an American Institution,* espoused the idea of individual planning in one of the major curricular recommendations: "Each student will have a Personal Plan for Progress to ensure that the high school takes individual needs into consideration . . ." (p. 11). More specifically related to transition, the document recommends that,

> By the time a student reaches the halfway point in high school, the Personal Plan for Progress should start emphasizing a transition plan to direct the student's curricular goals toward whatever it is that the young person wants to do after earning a diploma. Even a dropout will have a progress plan so that the youngster leaves with a blueprint for making as good use as possible of the immediate future and perhaps for returning to formal education. (p. 18)

Other guidelines could be offered—these are the ones that have been chosen for this book.

CHAPTER 3

School-Based Transition Practices

In this chapter, we present an overview of school-based practices related to providing transition services. The chapter is divided into two major sections. The first highlights current practices in assessment and planning and includes a model for understanding the sequence of moving from assessment to planning. The second focuses on the curricular implications of transition by looking at a number of instructional options. The very important aspect of linkage is addressed in Chapter 4.

TRANSITION ASSESSMENT AND PLANNING

Although the process of identifying transition needs and generating transition plans based on these needs is a relatively simple idea to present on a general level, the process gets much more complex as one looks closer. Figure 3.1 illustrates the key elements of this process. As can be seen in the figure, two immediate outcomes of assessment are possible: (1) recognition that more in-depth information is needed and (2) development of transition-related goals: knowledge and skills needs, which should be addressed through the development of instructional goals and subsequent instructional activities, and supports and services needs, which should be addressed through the generation of linkage goals and related activities to ensure that requisite connections are made. It is important to note that it is unlikely that both types of goals will be required for every transition area identified as needing attention.

Three themes seem to permeate the actual transition planning process and have significant implications on practice:

1. The more that is known about the receiving settings and the student's competence to deal with these settings, the more likely are the student's chances for success.
2. The more comprehensive the assessment of transition needs, the easier is the task of developing useful and appropriate transition plans.
3. The more the entire array of school-based professionals is involved in the transition process, the more likely they are to understand and be able to address a student's needs.

Transition Planning Areas

Although no set of transition planning areas has been agreed upon, it is possible to provide a sense of which planning areas are more frequently identified as critical for consideration. Table 3.1 shows the major transition domains identified in

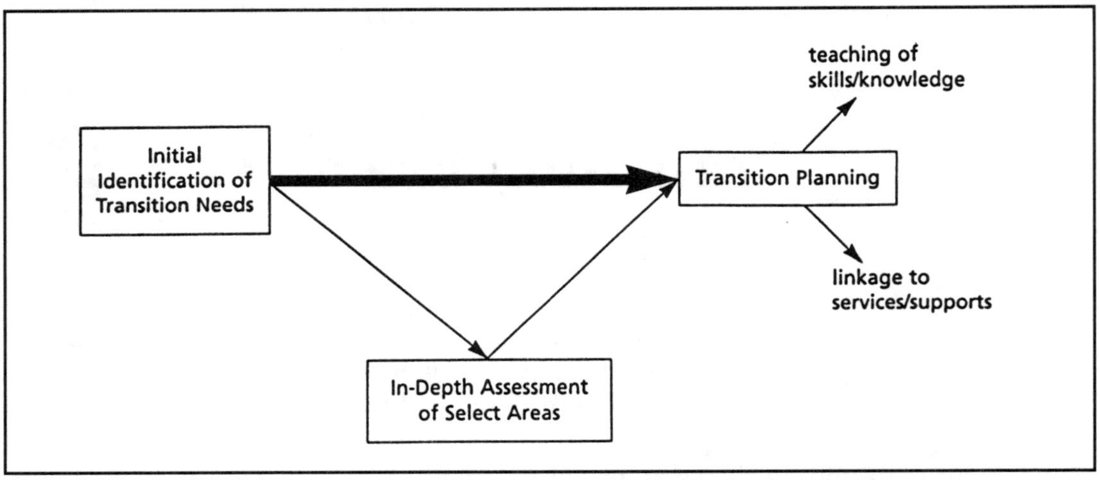

FIGURE 3.1. Transition planning process. From *Transition Planning Inventory* (p. 26), by G. M. Clark and J. R. Patton, 1997, Austin, TX: PRO-ED. Copyright 1997 by PRO-ED, Inc. Reprinted with permission.

the transition guides of 17 states. It should be noted that some states (e.g., Texas) embed certain planning areas within other domains. Although there is some degree of interstate variation, a common core of transition planning areas does emerge. Using the data provided in Table 3.1, the transition planning domains used by more than half of these states include the following (listed alphabetically):

- Community participation
- Daily living
- Employment
- Financial/income management
- Health
- Independent living (includes living arrangements)
- Leisure/recreation
- Postsecondary education
- Relationships/social skills
- Transportation/mobility
- Vocational training

Assessing Transition Needs

The collection of information about a student's transition needs requires a methodology that is useful for and easy to implement by school-based personnel. The importance of this task has been increased by the new requirement that a statement of transition needs be in place by age 14.

Many different methods and sources of information exist for generating a comprehensive picture of a student's transition needs. Table 3.2 provides a sampling of select commercially available techniques for acquiring transition planning information. Table 3.3 lists nonstandardized procedures that can provide useful information. For a more detailed discussion of assessment and various assess-

TABLE 3.1
Transition Planning Areas

Major Domains	States																
	AL	AR	CA	CO	CT	FL	HI	ID	IL	IA	KS	KY	LA	MN	NJ	TX	UT
Adult Services				X	X	X			X			X			X		
Advocacy/Legal	X							X					X				
Assistive Technology												X					
Career Planning Options								X									
Communication												X					X
Community Participation	X			X	X	X	X	X	X		X	X	X	X	X		X
Daily Living (including domestic areas)		X		X	X		X	X		X	X	X	X		X		X
Employment (including work-place readiness and specific job skills)	X	X	X	X	X	X		X	X	X	X	X	X		X	X	X
Financial/Income/Money Management	X		X		X		X	X		X	X	X	X				
Functional Academics															X		
Health (including medical services)	X			X	X		X	X		X	X	X	X		X		X
Independent Living (including living arrangements)	X	X	X		X	X		X	X		X	X	X	X	X	X	X
Insurance								X			X						
Leisure/Recreation		X	X	X	X		X	X		X	X	X	X	X	X	X	X
Lifelong Learning										X							
Personal Management	X																
Postsecondary Education		X	X	X	X	X	X	X	X		X	X	X	X	X	X	X
Relationships/Social Skills			X	X	X			X		X	X	X	X				X
Self-Determination/ Self-Advocacy					X			X		X	X	X		X			X
Transportation/Mobility	X	X		X	X		X	X		X	X	X	X		X		
Vocational Evaluation	X																
Vocational Training			X		X	X	X		X	X				X	X	X	X

Note. From *Transition Planning Inventory* (p. 4), by G. M. Clark and J. R. Patton, 1997, Austin, TX: PRO-ED. Copyright 1997 by PRO-ED, Inc. Reprinted with permission.

ment instruments, the reader is referred to Clark (1998) or Sitlington, Neubert, Begun, Lombard, and Leconte (1996).

Transition personnel need to know the features of the different instruments now available for determining transition needs. Furthermore, they must be able to locate and interpret existing assessment data. Most important, transition specialists must identify a system that allows them to identify the needs of many students quickly, yet comprehensively, so that sound transition plans can be developed.

TABLE 3.2

Commercially Available Tests and Procedures for Assessing Transition Needs

General Category	Selected Types of Measures	Specific Example(s)
Nonspecific to transition	Achievement tests	*Adult Basic Learning Examination–Second Edition* (Karlsen & Gardner, 1986)
	Adaptive behavior measures	*AAMR Adaptive Behavior Scales–School, Second Edition* (Lambert, Nihira, & Leland, 1993)
	Aptitude tests	*Differential Aptitude Test, Fifth Edition* (Bennett, Seashore, & Wesman, 1990)
	Communication tests	*Communicative Abilities in Daily Living* (Holland, 1980)
	Learning styles	*Learning Styles Inventory* (Dunn, Dunn, & Price, 1995)
	Manual dexterity	*Crawford Small Parts Dexterity Test* (Crawford, 1981)
	Occupational interest	*Occupational Aptitude Survey and Interest Schedule–2* (Parker, 1991)
	Personality/social skills	*Basic Personality Inventory* (Jackson, 1995)
Specific to transition	Needs assessment	*Transition Planning Inventory* (Clark & Patton, 1997) *Enderle–Severson Transition Rating Scale–Revised* (Enderle & Severson, 1997)
	Life skills	*BRIGANCE Life Skills Inventory* (Brigance, 1995) *LCCE Knowledge and Performance Battery* (Brolin, 1992) *Tests for Everyday Living* (Halpern, Irvin, & Landman, 1979)
	Self-determination	*Arc's Self-Determination Scale*
	Quality of life	*Quality of Life Questionnaire* (Schalock & Keith, 1993) *Quality of Student Life Questionnaire* (Keith & Schalock, 1995)
	Work-related behavior	*Transition Behavior Scale* (McCarney, 1989)
	Social	*Social and Prevocational Information Battery–Revised* (Halpern, Irvin, & Munkres, 1986)

TABLE 3.3

Types of Nonstandardized Assessment Instruments or Procedures, with Sample Items and Information

Instrument/Procedure	Sample Items/Information
Observational learning styles assessment	Student always goes to a quiet place to read. Student remembers things she sees.
Curriculum-based assessment (course specific)	Name the three branches of the federal government. What are two examples of toxic waste? Write a compound sentence.
Observational reports	J. C. complained of a headache twice today. M. N. needs help with grooming. O. P. gives no eye contact with girls.
Structured situational assessment	M. C. has been absent 10 days in 6 weeks. P. M. has been on time for work all month. J. P. completed every task assigned today. G. G. assembled 30 units with no errors.
Environmental assessment of student's situational placements or future placement options	M. C. is expected to prepare evening meals for five every evening at home. N. L. will be expected in algebra to compute probability problems. J. S. will be working in a work setting that is extremely high pressure and fast-paced.
Person-centered planning or futures planning procedures	What is your dream in life? What is your greatest fear of the future? Who are your best supports?
Structured interviews with students	What do you like to do with your free time? What are three occupations that interest you at this time?
Structured interviews with parents/ guardians	What would you like to see M. C. doing after she leaves school next year? Where and with whom would you like P. M. to live when he leaves home?
Social histories	M. C. has shown a consistent pattern of relating well to male authority figures. Since P. M.'s family moved and he went to live with his grandmother, he has run away from home six times. G. G. lives in a neighborhood that is high in drug-related activity and violence.

Note. From *Transition Planning Inventory* (p. 39), by G. M. Clark and J. R. Patton, 1997, Austin, TX: PRO-ED. Copyright 1997 by PRO-ED, Inc. Reprinted with permission.

Planning Based on Needs Assessment

For adequate plans to be developed, it is essential that a comprehensive needs assessment be conducted using a variety of sources and instrumentation. Equally important is the involvement of the student and his or her parents in the development of transition plans.

Types of Goals

Referring back to Figure 3.1, two types of outcomes, and therefore goal statements, should be generated from thorough transition planning: instructional activities and linkage activities. *Instructional goals* relate to knowledge and skills needs and should be written in the Individualized Education Program (IEP) as academic or social goals. For instance, if it is determined that a student needs to develop a specific study skill, such as note taking, to perform better in college, then an IEP goal should be written to address this need.

Linkage goals—the types of goals typically associated with transition planning—focus on making connections to the supports and services that will be needed in postschool situations and are written in the Individual Transition Plan (ITP) or the section of the IEP that deals with transition services. Continuing with the postsecondary education scenario referred to above, a college-bound student with disabilities could benefit from accessing the services of an office dedicated to working with students with special needs. A linkage goal should be written that ensures that the student is connected to this support service.

IEPs Versus ITPs

Some states require an ITP, which is a separate document from the IEP, as the principal vehicle for guiding transition activities. Other states simply include transition goals within the existing IEP under a section typically called "Statement of Transition Services." Both the ITP and the statement of transition services tend to include linkage types of goals.

Regardless of whether or not an ITP is used, the critical issue is that both knowledge/skills and linkage goal statements are generated for all areas of need. As mentioned earlier as one of the major themes, the actual individual planning phase is predicated on appropriate assessment procedures. The actual planning is easy if the assessment phase provides useful information across a range of transition planning areas.

Essential Elements of ITPs

The actual format of an ITP is not important, as long as goal statements for all areas needing instruction or linkage are listed. However, some ITP forms are better designed and organized than others. Most transition professionals will have to work with the forms their school districts have adopted until changes can be made.

Although great variation exists regarding ITP formats, every goal statement within the ITP should be accompanied by the following components:

- Present level of performance
- Specific activities needed to be performed to accomplish the goal
- Anticipated date of completion of activities
- Person(s) responsible

All of the components contribute to making this written document an important plan of action.

Most ITPs include other sections in addition to the goal statement section. Also, a section for a listing of persons participating in the ITP meeting is important. A sample ITP developed by Wehman (1995) is provided in Figure 3.2. All of the elements noted above can be found in this example. Additional information on developing transition plans can be found in Wehman (1998).

(text continues on page 33)

Student Profile

Krystal is a 17-year-old student who is approaching her last year at Eastland High School. She is enrolled in a LD class for one period a day. Most of her classes are in the regular classroom. Krystal leaves school for the last period of the day for 3 days a week to participate in student work experiences. Krystal is shy, but very likable. She is the oldest child of two and is part of a very supportive family who have always been very strong advocates for her.

Individual Transition Plan

Student's Name Krystal (First) ____ (M.I.) ____ (Last)

Birthdate ____ School Eastland High School

Student's ID No. ____ ITP Conference Date ____

Participants

Name	Position
Krystal	student
Miller	parent
Sadie	parent
Morris	special education teacher
Tim	rehabilitation counselor
Renée	classroom teacher

(continues)

Figure 3.2. Sample Individual Transition Plan. From *Individual Transition Plans: The Teacher's Curriculum Guide for Helping Youth with Special Needs* (pp. 139–144), by P. Wehman, 1995, Austin, TX: PRO-ED. Copyright 1995 by PRO-ED, Inc. Reprinted with permission.

I. Career and Economic Self-Sufficiency	
1. Employment Goal	Krystal will work in a hospital environment.
Level of present performance	Krystal has volunteered in a nursing home and has expressed an interest in a hospital environment upon exit from school.
Steps needed to accomplish goal	Krystal will (1) be given a full situational assessment of vocational activities; and (2) sample various jobs in a good hospital environment through career exploration.
Date of completion	7/95
Person(s) responsible for implementation	classroom teacher (lead person), rehabilitation counselor, and Krystal
2. Vocational Education/Training Goal	Krystal will learn skills specific to three positions in a hospital.
Level of present performance	Krystal has partial ability in cleaning and transporting skills. She also has shown interest in working in a hospital by performing volunteer work at a nursing home.
Steps needed to accomplish goal	Krystal will participate in student work experiences in a hospital environment to gain skills specific to the orderly, dietitian assistance, and registration desk positions.
Date of completion	6/95
Person(s) responsible for implementation	vocational coordinator (lead person), classroom teacher, student, and work experience coordinator
3. Postsecondary Education Goal	Krystal will enroll in an Allied Health Professional track at the community college.
Level of present performance	Krystal is enrolled in classes that teach skills in study habits and test taking in preparation for the Scholastic Aptitude Test (SAT). *(continues)*

Figure 3.2. *Continued.*

Steps needed to accomplish goal	Krystal needs to maintain a 2.5 grade point average and secure all Carnegie units to earn a high school diploma. She will study and take the SAT before she completes college entrance application.
Date of completion	9/95
Person(s) responsible for implementation	classroom teacher, Krystal, and parents
4. Financial/Income Needs Goal	Krystal will secure financial assistance to attend a community college program.
Level of present performance	Krystal is saving money in preparation for college in 1 year.
Steps needed to accomplish goal	Krystal will (1) secure various financial aid application packets; (2) complete and mail applications for financial aid; and (3) follow up with the college to verify benefits.
Date of completion	1/95
Person(s) responsible for implementation	parents, Krystal, and guidance counselor
II. Community Integration and Participation	
5. Independent Living Goal	Krystal will remain in home environment and continue to reside with parents while attending community college.
Level of present performance	Teacher will continue to facilitate discussions between the student and parents on the role of the student as a young adult living at home.
Steps needed to accomplish goal	Krystal will (1) identify ways to contribute to the household income; (2) discuss and agree with parents on the rules regarding house guests and curfews; and (3) use the family car.
Date of completion	9/94
Person(s) responsible for implementation	student, parents, and special education teacher

(*continues*)

Figure 3.2. *Continued.*

6. Transportation/Mobility Goal	N/A; Krystal has a driver's license.
Level of present performance	
Steps needed to accomplish goal	
Date of completion	
Person(s) responsible for implementation	
7. Social Relationships Goal	Krystal will develop one or more friendships with people in the neighborhood.
Level of present performance	Krystal is shy and does not usually approach others.
Steps needed to accomplish goal	Krystal will call Department of Recreation and Parks to inquire about the Teens Scene. She will acquire and complete an application and make arrangements to attend meetings.
Date of completion	9/95
Person(s) responsible for implementation	Krystal and parents
8. Recreation/Leisure Goal	Krystal will subscribe to Seventeen magazine.
Level of present performance	Krystal is concerned about teen issues such as health, safety, and leadership. Krystal enjoys reading and looking at fashion pictures.
Steps needed to accomplish goal	Teacher will help Krystal secure a subscription card to the magazine. Krystal will complete and mail the card. Krystal will access enough money from her savings account to pay for the magazines.

(continues)

Figure 3.2. *Continued.*

Date of completion	7/94
Person(s) responsible for implementation	Krystal, special education teacher, and parent
III. Personal Competence	
9. Health/Safety Goal	Krystal will access and understand information on building self-esteem and assertive communication.
Level of present performance	Although Krystal is shy, she has expressed an interest in participating in a program at the YWCA.
Steps needed to accomplish goal	Krystal will (1) find out when self-esteem/assertive communication class is offered; (2) she will sign up for classes; and (3) she will coordinate transportation with mother.
Date of completion	1/95
Person(s) responsible for implementation	special education teacher, parents, and Krystal
10. Self-Advocacy/Future Planning	Krystal will actively participate in discussions around graduation, college, work, independence, and money during the ITP meeting.
Level of present performance	Parents have always been strong advocates for Krystal.
Steps needed to accomplish goal	Krystal will be encouraged to ask questions and understand processes. She will be expected to actively participate in discussions about her transition plans.
Date of completion	6/95
Person(s) responsible for implementation	Krystal
Student Career Preference	
To work in a hospital	

(*continues*)

Figure 3.2. *Continued.*

Student's Major Transition Needs

1. Gain employment in hospital-related jobs
2. Participate in student work
3. Enroll in community college
4. Advocate for services
5. Participate more in social, recreational, and leisure programs
6.
7.
8.
9.

Additional Notes

Figure 3.2. *Continued.*

CURRICULAR IMPLICATIONS

The curriculum should be tied very closely to the issues surrounding transition. The fact that one of the goals of education is to prepare students to become contributing citizens implies that the content taught in school should have adult outcome referents. Furthermore, a major goal of the actual transition planning process is to determine needs, some of which will require instruction. Unfortunately, as Patton et al. (1997) pointed out, "consideration of specific content that must be taught to maximize students' chances for successfully dealing with the demands of adulthood and methods for teaching this content have been largely overlooked" (p. 299).

Instructional Models

Elements of transition education should be part of the educational programs of all students with special needs. A number of models exist that are helpful for providing instruction on topics closely related to adult outcomes. The similarities across the programs are numerous, as reflected in their materials, content taught, and types of suggested classroom activities. However, differences can typically be found, primarily in the way the curriculum is designed. This variance is not surprising, for as Armstrong (1989) noted, every curriculum design establishes a somewhat different set of priorities and provides for a program developed to respond to a particular set of needs determined or considered important by any number of individuals (e.g., teachers, parents, students, researchers, curriculum developers, community leaders). Most curricular models designed to prepare students for adult roles focus primarily on the introduction to and the acquisition of adult skills. Sitlington (1996) summarized a number of these models and their major components (see Table 3.4).

Instructional Considerations

Coverage of important life skills can be accomplished through either the establishment of coursework that is life skills/transition education oriented or the integration of life skills topics into existing content.

Life Skills Coursework Development

Cronin and Patton (1993) suggested several ways to organize life skills for instruction via adult outcome–oriented coursework. One method is to create a single course to cover multiple life skills topics (e.g., independent living skills or skills for life) as opposed to only one topic (e.g., English for work, functional math).

A more comprehensive approach is to create a series or set of life skills courses, with content and titles (e.g., personal finance, health and hygiene, and practical communications) based on situational needs. Helmke, Havekost, Patton, and Polloway (1994) described such an approach implemented by the Dubuque, Iowa, Community Schools.

Integration of Life Skills Topics into Existing Content

Another method of covering life skills topics is to augment existing courses and/or extend the coverage into more meaningful, life-related areas. In a consumer math course, for instance, a teacher might include additional lessons that address the

TABLE 3.4
Career Education and Life Skills Education Models

Source	Major Components
Life Centered Career Education (LCCE) (Brolin, 1993)	Three major areas: • Daily living • Personal–social • Occupational guidance and preparation
School-Based Career Development and Transition Education Model (Clark & Kolstoe, 1995)	Four major areas: • Values, attitudes, and habits • Human relationships • Occupational information • Acquisition of job and daily living skills
Hawaii Transition Project (University of Hawaii, 1987)	Four major areas: • Vocation/education • Home and family • Recreation/leisure • Community/citizenship
Community-Referenced Curriculum (Smith & Schloss, 1988)	Five major areas: • Work • Leisure and play • Consumer • Education and rehabilitation • Transportation
Community Living Skills Taxonomy (Dever, 1988)	Five major areas: • Personal maintenance and development • Homemaking and community life • Vocational • Leisure • Travel
Life Problems of Adulthood (Knowles, 1990)	Six major areas: • Vocation and career • Home and family living • Enjoyment of leisure • Community living • Health • Personal development
Domains of Adulthood (Cronin & Patton, 1993)	Six major areas: • Employment/education • Home and family • Leisure pursuits • Community involvement • Physical/emotional health • Personal responsibility and relationships
Post-School Outcomes Model (National Center on Educational Outcomes, 1993)	Seven major areas: • Presence and participation • Physical health • Responsibility and independence • Contribution and citizenship • Academic and functional literacy • Personal and social adjustment • Satisfaction
Quality of Life Domains (Halpern, 1993)	Three major areas: • Physical and material well-being • Performance of adult roles • Personal fulfillment

Note. From "Transition to Living: The Neglected Components of Transition Programming for Individuals with Learning Disabilities," by P. L. Sitlington, 1996, *Journal of Learning Disabilities, 29,* p. 35. Copyright 1996 by PRO-ED, Inc. Reprinted with permission.

life skills associated with moving into an apartment. For many students, this might be a particularly important life demand that is not typically covered in secondary school instructional materials.

In the infusion approach, the objective is to infuse into existing courses life skill topics that relate directly to information being covered. This approach requires close examination of course content to establish whether important life skills that students will need as adults are being covered.

This approach infuses relevance into course content taught on a daily basis in addition to covering life skills topics, no matter what the subject of the class might be. Further, this approach may be the only one available for students in inclusive settings. It gives relevance to the content being taught to both students identified as disabled and their nondisabled peers.

CHAPTER 4

Postsecondary Considerations: A Need for Linkage

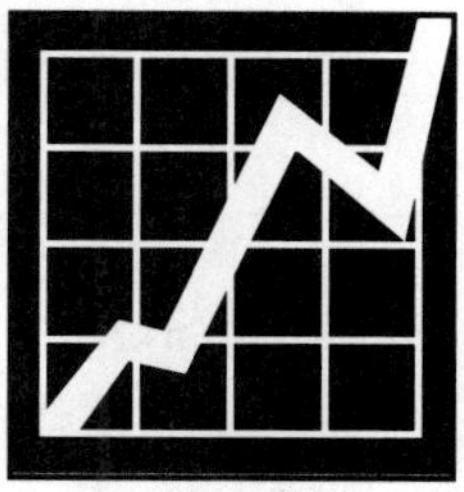

A question that many educators, parents, and individuals with disabilities ask themselves during the transition planning and program development process is "transition from school to what?" The answer to this question can vary dramatically from individual to individual, depending on a variety of factors, including the individual's interests, abilities, and local community. For example, the "what" might be attending a university in another city and living in a college dormitory; or job training at a community trade or technical school and living at home; or employment and living with a friend; or supported employment and living in a small group home. Many individuals with disabilities might need assistance with time management and budgeting, and perhaps some would need counseling and self-advocacy training. What is important to recognize is that there is a wide range of postsecondary considerations for transition planning. Planning for transition involves more than employment training; comprehensive planning considers the range of adult roles an individual will eventually assume. This chapter begins with an overview of the kinds of postsecondary linkages that are available. A discussion of the primary service providers in the transition process and the need for interagency collaboration among service providers follows.

POSTSECONDARY AREAS OF FOCUS

Employment/Nonemployment

Employment is an important part in the lives of all individuals. The kind of job one has, the amount of money one makes, and the opportunities that are available for advancement affect not only how society views the individual but also how the individual views him- or herself (Wehman, Moon, Everson, Wood, & Barcus, 1988). Thus, one of the primary postsecondary linkage considerations for students with disabilities is employment.

An array of employment options for individuals with disabilities exists, ranging from nonemployment to competitive employment (see Table 4.1). These options vary on several dimensions, including whether the individual receives financial reimbursement, the kinds of employment supports provided, and the degree of community integration (Beirne-Smith, Ittenbach, & Patton, 1998; Schutz, 1988; Vogelsberg & Schutz, 1988). Determining the option that is best for an individual at a given point in time is a function of the interaction of a number of factors, including economic conditions, extent and adequacy of training, characteristics of the employment site, and characteristics of the individual (Beirne-Smith et al., 1998). A brief description of each of the options is presented below.

TABLE 4.1

Employment Options for Individuals with Disabilities

Employment Option	Example/Explanation	Dimension: Financial Reimbursement	Dimension: Employment Supports	Dimension: Community Integration
Nonemployment	• Individual's need for supports so pervasive that employment is unlikely • Individual chooses not to work • Individual cannot find work	No	No	No
Unpaid	• Volunteer work	No	Varies	Likely
Paid: Sheltered	• Adult day programs • Work activity centers • Sheltered workshops	Below minimum	Continual	No
Paid: Supported	• Individual placement • Enclave • Mobile work crew • Benchwork • Entrepreneurial	Minimum or higher	Continual/ faded	Yes
Paid: Competitive	• Full- or part-time jobs in open labor market	Minimum or higher	Varies	Yes

Note. Adapted from *Mental Retardation* (5th ed., p. 400), by M. Beirne-Smith, R. Ittenbach, and J. Patton, 1998, New York: Prentice-Hall/Merrill Education.

Nonemployment

There are three primary reasons why an individual might not be employed (Beirne-Smith et al., 1998). One reason is that the individual's needs for supports are so pervasive or the individual has such limited skills that vocational training leading to employment is unlikely. A second reason for nonemployment is that an individual who is capable of working chooses not to. Some individuals prefer nonemployment simply because they do not want to work, whereas others choose nonemployment because of disincentives for working, such as loss of medical and health benefits. Finally, some individuals have the skills and desire to work, but cannot find employment.

Unpaid Employment

Unpaid employment refers to work without financial compensation. For some individuals, working without pay can be viewed as a positive situation because the individual is involved in an ongoing activity and income is not expected (Beirne-Smith et al., 1998). An example of this is volunteer work. For others, the benefits of having access to the same kinds of employment options as those without disabilities and inclusion in nonrestrictive settings outweigh paid employment in a restrictive setting (L. Brown et al., 1984).

Paid Employment

There are three main options for paid employment, ranging from employment in highly protected and segregated settings to employment in highly competitive and integrated settings.

Sheltered Employment. In a sheltered employment setting, individuals with disabilities who require constant supervision work in a self-contained unit, with no integration with workers without disabilities. Sheltered employment options range from adult day programs to work activity centers to sheltered workshops and are typically supported by federal and/or state funds (National Information Center for Children and Youth with Disabilities [NICHCY], 1991). The focus of *adult day programs* is usually on daily living skills, social skills, recreational skills, and prevocational skills training. *Work activity centers* address these same skills, but they also provide vocational skills training. In *sheltered workshops,* individuals generally perform jobs or tasks that have been subcontracted, such as packaging, collating, sewing, or machine assembly. Workers are usually paid on a piece-rate basis.

Supported Employment. Supported employment is for individuals with severe disabilities who need ongoing support services to perform competitive work in integrated settings. The element that distinguishes this approach from others is the provision of ongoing support (NICHCY, 1991). In supported employment, the individual with a disability is provided with the support necessary to learn and maintain a job. Employment support continues indefinitely, although the amount of support needed typically decreases over time.

There are five general types of supported employment models. It should be noted, however, that elements from several of the models are combined in many communities (NICHCY, 1991). In the *individual placement* model, the individual with a disability receives intensive one-on-one job training from a job coach until a specified level of proficiency is attained, at which time the amount of support is gradually decreased. In the *enclave* model, a small group of individuals with disabilities is trained and supervised alongside employees without disabilities by a human services professional or an employee of the company. The *mobile work crew* model is characterized by a group of 4 to 6 individuals with disabilities who move from business to business providing services such as cleaning or lawn care. The crew is accompanied by a supervisor or manager who is responsible for the training and supervision of the workers. In the *benchwork* model, contract work is obtained from electronics firms and related industries. A group of 8 to 15 workers with disabilities are then trained and supervised by a small number of qualified staff. The *entrepreneurial* model is characterized by workers with and without disabilities working at a not-for-profit job site. Supervision is usually provided by human service workers.

Competitive Employment. Competitive employment is defined as "full-time or part-time jobs in the open labor market with competitive wages and responsibilities" (NICHCY, 1991, p. 5). The individual with a disability does not receive any more outside support than co-workers without a disability would receive with regard to job maintenance. However, the individual with a disability might have participated in a transitional job training and placement program in order to obtain the job. The amount of support provided prior to employment will vary depending on the individual's needs and abilities. Some might need assistance only with locating a job, whereas others will need extensive vocational training. Still others might need to explore postsecondary academic opportunities necessary for their career choice. The critical difference between this model and the supported employment model is that, in the competitive work model, assistance and support are time limited and cease after the person has obtained employment.

Postsecondary Education and Training

For some, employment is not an immediate postsecondary goal. Rather, these individuals might choose to continue employment preparation and career development beyond high school through participation in postsecondary academic and vocational programs. Both formal and informal postsecondary training alternatives exist for individuals with disabilities. Postsecondary academic programs include 4-year college/university and graduate degree programs, whereas postsecondary vocational programs include all programs that do not grant degrees at the bachelor's level or higher, such as 2-year community college programs and trade and business schools (Gajar, Goodman, & McAfee, 1993). Table 4.2 summarizes key information concerning academic and vocational programs. Other postsecondary education and training opportunities include job training programs, military service, and functional academic skill building. A brief discussion of these is provided below.

Academic Programs

The number of students with disabilities pursuing postsecondary education is increasing due to the recognition that some individuals with disabilities can benefit from and be successful in such programs. There are several reasons why a student might attend a postsecondary academic program. For some students, the completion of a 4-year program will hopefully lead to an entry-level career job. For others, a college degree might be a stepping stone to advanced graduate or professional training (Scheiber & Talpers, 1987). This option is most appropriate for students with mild disabilities who have higher IQs and academic skill levels (Minskoff, 1994). Academic programs typically provide accommodations, such as recorded reading materials, untimed exams, study skills training, and self- and time-management skill development for individuals with disabilities (Gajar et al., 1993). Some colleges and universities provide additional services, including developmental year programs, tutoring, personal or social counseling, academic or program counseling, or career and vocational counseling. The latter part of the Appendix includes a listing of guides and resources for identifying postsecondary academic programs for individuals with disabilities.

Vocational Programs

Vocational training can be acquired through 2-year college programs, vocational education, and other training programs.

Two-Year Colleges. Both public and private community and junior colleges provide students with the opportunity to try out postsecondary education. This alternative provides many students with the occasion to prepare for further education or learn an occupational skill (Scheiber & Talpers, 1987). For others, this option provides a means for personal development. Upon completion of a 2-year program, students earn an Associate of Arts (AA) degree. Credits can be transferred to 4-year colleges or universities. Courses of study in specific occupations, such as child care or bookkeeping, usually take less than 2 years to complete and result in a certificate.

Vocational Education. Vocational education is "education geared for employment that requires specialized education but not a baccalaureate (BA) degree" (Scheiber & Talpers, 1987, p. 51). It can provide the student with professional training necessary for the development of marketable skills and a job future.

(text continues on page 45)

TABLE 4.2

Postsecondary Education and Training Options

Option	Dimension			
	Admission Requirements	**Emphasis**	**General Information**	**Outcome**
Colleges, Universities	***Regular*** High school diploma or GED SAT or ACT GPA and/or class rank ***Special or Provisional*** SAT/ACT may be waived or lower scores accepted Other factors (e.g., potential, goals) considered Remedial or study skills classes may be required ***Cooperative (special program within college)*** Joint decision between college and special program Must disclose disability Some require ACT/SAT Some require high school diploma/GED	4-year program Extensive selection of majors (>400) Sample a variety of courses during first 2 years Select major in last 2 years Some colleges specialize (music, design, technology)	Tuition varies greatly State-supported generally less costly Financial aid usually available Several sources of help available (counseling, peer tutoring, learning labs, math centers)	Bachelor of Science Degree, Bachelor of Arts Degree

(continues)

TABLE 4.2 *Continued.*

Option	Dimension: Admission Requirements	Emphasis	General Information	Outcome
Community and Junior Colleges, Public, 2-Year	Usually open admission 18 years or older Most require high school diploma or GED for credit courses	2-year program Liberal arts subjects Training in specific occupations (hotel management, auto mechanics, marketing, dental hygiene) Many also have remedial or developmental courses for upgrading basic academic skills Provides student with opportunity to try out college by taking one or two courses	Available in or near most cities Less expensive than 4-year programs Committed to serving educational and training needs of local communities Provides opportunity to build a better academic record that can be transferred to a 4-year program Provides opportunity to upgrade academic and job skills and work toward improved employment opportunities or a career change	Associates of Arts Degree, Certificate in Specific Occupations
Junior Colleges, Private, 2-Year	High school diploma or GED Usually an entrance exam (SAT or ACT) Usually request GPA and/or class rank Experience and personal qualities usually considered	General course of study Prepares students to transfer to a 4-year liberal arts institution Opportunities to improve reading, writing, and math skills Opportunities to train for a new career	Most are small, residential schools Small class sizes Individualized attention	Associates of Arts Degree

(*continues*)

TABLE 4.2 *Continued.*

Option	Admission Requirements	Emphasis	General Information	Outcome
	Dimension			
Vocational Education Schools, Public and Private, 2 Years or Less	Usually open admission Some require high school diploma or GED Some require SAT, ACT, or admission tests	***Community Junior Colleges*** Occupational training and liberal arts training can be combined ***2-Year Technical Institutes/Colleges*** Degree programs in skill areas needed to enter and advance in specific occupational fields Academic courses usually related to occupational areas ***Area Vocational Centers or Single-Specialty Public Vocational and Technical Schools*** Available in a few areas Offer training in a single-specialty skill (e.g., aviation, truck driving, barbering) ***Private*** Trade, technical, or business schools Offers training in a variety of occupational skills Practical training in fields requiring 2 years or less	Great variability in patterns of service due to the state laws that govern (e.g., some states may offer vocational education through the community college system, whereas others might offer through technical institutes) Also great variability in state requirements for licenses to practice trades and courses of study to complete programs	Associate of Arts, Certificate

Note. Adapted from *Unlocking Potential: College and Other Choices for Learning Disabled People. A Step-by-Step Guide* (pp. 46–47, 53–56, 81), by B. Scheiber & J. Talpers, 1987, Bethesda, MD: Adler & Adler.

Vocational education programs are available in public and private institutions. Examples of public programs include area vocational centers, community colleges, and technical institutes. Trade, technical, and business schools are examples of private programs. Vocational education programs teach occupational skills in a wide range of areas, including agriculture/agribusiness, marketing and distributing, health, business and office, trade and industry, and occupational home economics. The length of time required to complete a vocational program varies from 10 weeks to 2 years, depending on the occupational requirements of the area and the skill level to be attained. Upon completion of the program, students receive either a degree or a certificate. Completion of a 2-year course of technical training in an occupational area usually leads to an Associate of Applied Science (AAS) or an Associate of Applied Arts (AAA) degree, whereas completion of specific occupational skill training leads to a certificate. Although certificate programs have the same requirements for mastery of occupational skills as degree programs, the former do not require the same amount of academic coursework, taking 1 year or less to complete (Scheiber & Talpers, 1987). In some fields, such as plumbing and nursing, the individual must be licensed, which requires the student to do additional work after completing a degree or certificate program. See the Appendix for resources identifying vocational training programs.

Other Postsecondary Education and Training Opportunities

In addition to the traditional college, university, and vocational educational programs, a variety of other options are available to assist individuals with disabilities to acquire job skills, job training, and related academic skills. Some of these training programs are available while the individual is in high school. Some options are available for both individuals with and without disabilities, whereas others are specific options available only to those with disabilities. Many of these programs, however, are in short supply, and thus may be difficult to locate (Scheiber & Talpers, 1987).

Tech Prep. Tech Prep, authorized by the Carl D. Perkins Act of 1990, is actually a combined secondary and postsecondary program. It is a 4-year sequence of study that prepares students for a highly skilled technical occupation that allows either (a) direct entry into the workplace as a qualified technician or (b) continuation with further education leading to baccalaureate and advanced degrees. Students begin the course of study in their junior year of high school and complete it after 2 years of postsecondary occupational education that culminates in a certificate or associate degree. Information about Tech Prep programs can be obtained from the State Vocational and Adult Education Office or the Office of Vocational and Adult Education, U.S. Department of Education.

On-the Job Training Program (OJT). On-the-job training is short-term training that allows an individual to work on a job site while learning the job duties from a supervisor or co-worker. The trainee may or may not be paid, but the training has the possibility of leading to the trainee's assuming the job as an employee of the company in which he or she is being trained. In this approach, the employers providing the OJT are supported with services or monetary incentives. This training approach is used by many different programs, including the State Vocational Rehabilitation (VR) program and Job Training Partnership Act programs. OJT is also available for individuals with disabilities from some large companies such as IBM, which runs its program in cooperation with the National Technical Institute for the Deaf and Gallaudet University, and disability organizations such as the Arc, which has a national OJT program that locates jobs for individuals with mental retardation. Information about OJT programs can be obtained through the State Office of Vocational Rehabilitation, State Employment Offices, or organizations such as the Arc.

Job Training Partnership Act (JTPA). Another source of employment training opportunities is through the Job Training Partnership Act. The purpose of JTPA-funded programs is to prepare youth and unskilled adults for entry into the labor market (NICHCY, 1991). JTPA programs are funded by the federal government and run locally by a Private Industry Council (PIC). PICs include representatives of local businesses, education agencies, and state and local governments. Examples of services provided through local training programs include preemployment training, job counseling, vocational training, remedial education and basic-skills training, job placement assistance, work experience, and literacy and bilingual training. Funds for summer youth employment programs also are available through JTPA. Target populations include individuals who are economically disadvantaged and others who face serious barriers to employment, including individuals with disabilities. Information about JTPA programs can be obtained from local employment agencies, human services agencies that provide training in the area in which the individual is interested, or the state JTPA liaison person.

Projects with Industry (PWI). Projects with Industry are federally financed cooperative arrangements between business, industry, and rehabilitation services (C. Brown & Browning, 1997). The link in this partnership is a business advisory council. The purpose of PWIs is to promote opportunities for individuals with disabilities to attain competitive employment through the involvement of private industry. The availability of such programs varies from community to community. Information about local PWI programs can be obtained from the state VR agency.

Training Offered by Disability-Specific Organizations. Organizations serving individuals with a specific disability, such as the Arc, United Cerebral Palsy, and others, may provide vocational assessment and training. For example, many regional offices of the Arc offer computer skills and other office skills training to persons with mental retardation who have been referred to their office. This training has frequently led to competitive employment. Although the types of training vary, the goals of the programs are similar—striving to assist the individual to obtain employment and become as independent as possible (NICHCY, 1991). Information about such programs can be obtained from the local, state, or national office of the organization.

Community Rehabilitation Programs (CRPs). Another job training option for students exiting high school is through Community Rehabilitation Programs or Centers. These programs are typically provided by the state VR agency. CRPs provide services in prevocational development, job training, and adult basic education. The recent emphases on inclusion and consumer-driven approaches, however, have resulted in criticism of this option because the services and training are provided in segregated settings (Brown & Browning, 1997). Consequently, many of these programs have experienced dramatic changes in the past few years. Contact the state VR agency for information about the availability of these programs.

Internship and Apprenticeship Programs. Internships are similar to OJT in that they are time limited and can be paid or unpaid employment. They allow the individual to sample the kind of work available in a general area (NICHCY, 1991). Many high schools and community employment training programs use this kind of experience. In an apprenticeship program, an individual, who is hired at an entry level, learns a craft or trade by working under the supervision of an experienced supervisor. These programs usually take 3 to 4 years to complete. Beginning wages are often near minimum wage, but toward the end of the program, the individuals are frequently earning wages near those of experienced workers. There are over 700 occupations for which apprenticeship programs exist. Information about apprenticeship programs can be obtained from local unions, vocational education programs in the community, state departments of labor, and state offices of vocational rehabilitation.

Military Service. The highly structured and physically active nature of the military is a viable option for some individuals with disabilities (Scheiber & Talpers, 1987). Military training consists of both classroom work and field experiences. Military service can lead to employment or additional education at the college level. Individuals must take the Armed Services Vocational Aptitude Battery prior to enlisting in the armed forces. This battery assesses reading, spelling, math, general, and mechanical knowledge. It screens out those who are not able to perform adequately in basic skill areas.

Adult Education. Adult education includes a wide variety of learning opportunities for individuals who are not in high school, including courses designed to help students obtain a high school diploma and learn functional literacy skills (Scheiber & Talpers, 1987). *Adult basic education* (ABE) programs focus on basic educational skills necessary for employment and meeting adult responsibilities for individuals with learning deficits, limited English language proficiency, or physical or mental disabilities. The federal government provides the funding for ABE programs to state and counties. Priority is given to those with the lowest literacy skills. Every state has a department of adult education; information about local ABE programs can be obtained from local education agencies. *Literacy groups* across the country also provide adult education. These groups are usually staffed by trained volunteers who work one-on-one with a student. In general, the literacy training is not geared toward those with disabilities; however, recently there has been an increased recognition of the number of individuals with disabilities participating in such programs.

Residential and Leisure Arrangements

Various residential options exist for individuals with disabilities, ranging from independent living to small group homes to large, public facilities. The importance of where one lives cannot be ignored because where people live determines to a great extent how they live (Beirne-Smith et al., 1998). Residence influences where the person can work and the community services and resources that are available, as well as friendships (Heward, 1996). Additionally, recreation and leisure activities have assumed a prioritized and expanding role in the lives of Americans (Wehman, 1979). However, this area is often neglected, even though participation in recreation and leisure activities plays an integral role in community adjustment (Schleien, Rynders, & Green, 1994). Similar to other linkage considerations, various recreation and leisure options are available for individuals with disabilities.

Residential Alternatives

Over the years a marked shift has occurred from residential to community settings. The residential options available to individuals with disabilities can be viewed along a continuum from integrated services that require a high degree of independence or support to segregated services that tend to foster dependence (Clees, 1992). Table 4.3 provides a summary of these options.

Most professionals agree that no single residential setting is best for individuals with disabilities, and that there is a need for a continuum of options (Heward, 1996). Some, however, have concerns about the continuum-of-services approach as it relates to residential options. A major concern is that most continuum-of-service models are based on the assumption that an individual begins the residential service system at the more restrictive end; the individual must then earn the right to less restrictive living alternatives. Some have argued instead that residential placements must be adapted to meet the needs of the individual with a disability (Klein, 1994). The term *supported living* has been used to describe this type of placement. Discussed next are the major categories of residential alternatives.

Independent Living. An individual is considered to be living independently only if he or she is not receiving any supports other than what are typically available to those without disabilities (Clees, 1992). Independent living can include living with a roommate, a spouse, or alone, in an apartment, duplex, or house. Such arrangements range from single-family homes to individual or shared apartments to residential hotels.

Supported Living in Own Apartment or Home. Supported living is much like supported employment in that the individual is provided with ongoing support. In supported living, individuals are enabled to "receive the support they need and to live in a home they want" (Klein, 1994, p. 18). Semi-independent living services (SILS) enable an individual to live in the community with supports. These individuals are those who might otherwise live in a more restrictive setting. Support services include training, counseling, and assistance in areas of independent living (e.g., financial management, grocery shopping, medical issues). Such services are often available through the county. Personal care assistant services are coordinated through independent living services provided by Vocational Rehabilitation and are appropriate for individuals who need assistance with physical health or care issues (e.g., medication administration, bladder care, range of motion, positioning).

Protected Settings. Protected settings provide varying amounts of support and supervision to individuals with disabilities. The goal of these options is to permit the individual to live as completely and independently as possible in a family-oriented setting (Beirne-Smith et al., 1998). The use of *foster homes* for adults with disabilities is increasing. In a foster home setting, a family opens up its home to an unrelated person for an extended period of time. The family usually provides room and board, for which it receives a modest financial reimbursement. An increasing number of individuals with disabilities are participating in *apartment living* alternatives. This option provides an even greater opportunity for community integration than group homes (Heward, 1996). In an *apartment cluster* option, a small number of apartments house individuals with disabilities, while a supervisor lives in a nearby apartment. A *co-residence apartment* option is when an individual with disability has a roommate without a disability.

Group Homes. Supervised living in a group home is another residential option. Group homes are small community-based homes for fewer than 16 residents. They are the fastest growing residential option for adults with mental retardation, providing family-style living (Heward, 1996). In these homes, groups of individuals with disabilities, usually 3 to 6, live in a residential neighborhood. Live-in coun-

TABLE 4.3
Residential Options

Option	Examples	Description
Independent living	Single-family home Shared home (two or more individuals with disabilities) Apartment	No support other than what is typically available to those without disabilities Alone or with a roommate or spouse
Supported living in own apartment or home	Semi-independent living services (e.g., training and assistance with financial management or grocery shopping) provided in own home or apartment Personal care assistant services (e.g., assistance with medication administration, bladder care) provided in own home or apartment	Services provided to enable an individual, who might otherwise live in a more restrictive setting, to live in a home or apartment of his or her own
Protected settings	Foster homes Apartment living	Varying amounts of support and supervision provided Goal is to allow the individual to live as completely and independently as possible
Group homes	Residential (i.e., permanent) Transitional (i.e., short term)	Small community-based homes for fewer than 16 people Live-in counselors supervise and support
Large group facilities	Intermediate care facilities–mental retardation Nursing homes Institutions or developmental centers	Fully staffed residential facilities 16 or more residents (average size is >300 people)

selors supervise and support the residents. Some homes are *residential,* representing a permanent or long-term living arrangement for the individual, whereas others are *transitional,* preparing the individual for a more independent living situation.

Large Group Facilities. Large residential facilities are defined as serving 16 or more residents. The average size of most large residential facilities, however, is greater than 300 people (Heward, 1996). The number of individuals living in large group facilities has decreased in recent decades. Residential living, however, is still chosen for some with disabilities, particularly those with severe mental retardation and multiple disabilities. *Intermediate care facilities–Mental retardation* (ICF-MR) are facilities that are licensed as nursing homes, which makes them eligible for federal Medicaid support. *State-supported institutions* are fully staffed residential facilities providing services to 16 or more individuals with disabilities. *Nonstate-supported institutions* are also fully staffed facilities providing services to 16 or more individuals with disabilities; however, they are operated privately or by the local government. *Nursing homes* are another large group facility option. Medical, nursing, and personal care are provided to individuals with and without disabilities.

Recreation and Leisure Alternatives

There are many benefits of participation in recreation and leisure activities, including physical health and conditioning, development and expansion of skill repertoires, expansion of social networks, development of a more positive self-concept, and establishment of a more fulfilling way of life (Schleien et al., 1994). It has only been within the last 15 years that this area has received consideration. Sources for information on recreation and leisure programs for individuals with disabilities are listed in the Appendix.

Segregated Recreation Programs. Segregated programs are those specifically designed for individuals with disabilities and in which only those with disabilities participate.

Integration of Generic Recreation Programs. Integration of a generic recreation program is when individuals with disabilities are included in existing recreation programs. Individuals with disabilities are supported in selecting an existing age-appropriate community recreation program; a support person then works with the generic recreation program leader to address the discrepancies between the program skill requirements and the individual's skills (Schleien et al., 1994).

Reverse Mainstreaming. In reverse mainstreaming, segregated programs for individuals with disabilities are modified to attract individuals without disabilities. An example of this approach is Special Olympics International's Unified Sports Team, in which approximately the same number of individuals with and without mental retardation are on the same team. Unified Sports leagues have been established nationwide for basketball, bowling, soccer, softball, and volleyball.

Zero Exclusion Team Approach. In the zero exclusion team approach, therapeutic recreation specialists and generic recreation program leaders collaboratively plan an activity prior to its implementation. The assumption is made that new programs will include individuals both with and without disabilities.

Community and Daily Living Needs

A final postsecondary linkage consideration is community and daily living needs. The identification of postsecondary training and education and residential alternatives is much easier than the identification of community and daily living needs (Clark & Kolstoe, 1995). Further, training in community and daily living areas is often "left to chance or presumed to be best suited for informal training and incidental learning" (Clark & Kolstoe, 1995, p. 360). Many individuals with disabilities, however, will need assistance in these areas. Listed below are training sources.

Colleges and Universities

In addition to academic or vocational classes, many colleges and universities provide counseling or mental health services, as well as opportunities for personal–social development, including group problem-solving meetings, guest lectures on adjustment to college, and noncredit seminars or workshops on selected topics such as problem drinking, depression, recreational drug use, sexuality, suicide, or health-related topics (Clark & Kolstoe, 1995). Further, credit courses that address personal development and human adjustment are frequently offered.

Adult Education

Adult education can provide an opportunity for skill development in independent living areas. For example, courses in such areas as cooking, auto mechanics, woodworking, consumer education, and introduction to microcomputers are often available through adult education (Clark & Kolstoe, 1995).

Independent Living Centers (ILCs) and Independent Living Programs

The specific intent of *independent living centers* is to address problems in independent living and personal–social adjustment. These programs assist individuals in learning how to take charge of their lives at home and in the community in multiple areas, including emotional, social, vocational, and daily living. Independent living centers evolved from self-help groups that were established by individuals with disabilities (Jones & Ulciny, 1986). The centers are community-based, nonprofit, nonresidential programs that are controlled by the individuals with disabilities. The key features that distinguish them from other kinds of independent living programs are (a) consumer involvement at all levels of decision making, (b) focus on individualized services for individuals with disabilities, and (c) focus on community change efforts (Jones & Ulciny, 1986). ILCs are diverse in organization, management, and types of services provided.

Other kinds of *independent living programs* have been developed to address the area of independent living. Such programs focus primarily on teaching skills necessary for living independently in the community and obtaining and maintaining employment. Some of these programs are residential. Unlike ILCs, these programs are usually run by professionals. The Appendix includes resources on independent living programs.

Mental Health Centers

Individuals classified as having behavioral disorders or mild mental retardation tend to need mental health services more than those with other disabilities (Clark & Kolstoe, 1995). Mental health centers serve those with severe personal, social, or adjustment difficulties, providing individual or group counseling.

TRANSITION SERVICE PROVIDERS AND NEED FOR INTERAGENCY COLLABORATION

Although educators play a critical role in preparing students for future work, education/training, residential, and community environments, they do not have the time or the ability to accomplish these outcomes on their own (Blalock, 1996). The successful transition from secondary to postsecondary environments is the shared responsibility of many, because the very nature and complexity of the process is such that neither teachers, "families, schools, adult service providers, state agencies, nor post-secondary institutions can carry the entire fiscal, programmatic or [transition] planning responsibility" (National Transition Network, 1993a, p. 3).

While the student is at the secondary level, school personnel serve as coordinator or case manager for educational and vocational programs, and services are provided in a fairly organized manner (NICHCY, 1991). Upon exiting the school system, however, the individual works with an array of service providers with differing eligibility requirements. As such, there is no longer a single agency responsible for coordinating and providing services. To ensure that a smooth transition occurs from secondary to postsecondary environments, it is imperative that school personnel are familiar with the major service systems available for assisting in the transition process. This information not only helps in the development of a comprehensive transition program while the student is in school, but also helps to ensure that the student moves immediately into postsecondary programs upon graduation.

The concept of interagency cooperation and collaboration is highlighted in federal legislation drafted in the 1990s. Although the core legislation for this partnership is in special education (the Individuals with Disabilities Education Act), legislation in vocational education (Carl D. Perkins Vocational and Applied Technology Education Act Amendments of 1990), rehabilitation (Rehabilitation Act Reauthorization of 1992), and other areas "provides clear evidence that transition preparation must extend beyond the school walls, and thus become a multishared responsibility among various players, disciplines, and programs" (Brown & Browning, 1997).

Special Education

A key characteristic of special education is that it is an entitlement program. What this means is that all students who have a disability that interferes with their ability to benefit from general education services are guaranteed a free, appropriate public education. Also, special education operates from a single agency and legislative act (Everson, 1993). With respect to transition, the Individuals with Disabilities Education Act (IDEA) mandates the provision of a coordinated set of transition activities within an outcome-oriented process for *all* students with disabilities. Beginning at age 14, a statement of transition service needs that focuses on the student's course of study must be included in the IEP. Beginning at age 16, a statement of needed transition services must be included in the IEP. Further, IDEA requires that interagency linkages be established to increase the effectiveness of service delivery while the student is in school and to support his or her movement to postsecondary settings. Although the public agency (usually the school) is primarily responsible for the provision of transition services, IDEA clearly signals that preparing students to move from school to postschool environments is not the sole responsibility of public education. During the transition planning process, educators, parents, and personnel from other programs and agencies should coordinate the secondary coursework, work experiences, community participation, and home responsibilities necessary to prepare the student for postsecondary linkages (Dowdy & Evers, 1996). Further, the responsibilities of participating agencies or postsecondary linkages for a given student must be designated before the student leaves school.

Vocational Education

Vocational education is designed to assist individuals with and without disabilities to develop specific occupational skills through sequential educational instruction and training appropriate for each individual's skills and abilities. Its overall goal is to provide vocational education to develop fundamental, academic, and employability skills for employment in the individual's vocational area of interest

(Dowdy & Evers, 1996). Vocational education funds support both secondary and postsecondary programs. Some of the linkage considerations discussed earlier in this section are supported with vocational education monies.

With regard to transition, one of the assurances of the Carl D. Perkins Vocational and Applied Technology Education Act Amendments of 1990 is that there is coordination among appropriate representatives of vocational education, special education, and vocational rehabilitation. Section 403.190(b)(1) and (5) of the act requires that recipients of Perkins funds (a) assist eligible students with disabilities in fulfilling the transition service requirements of Section 626 of IDEA and (b) provide counseling and instructional services designed to facilitate the transition from school to work.

Adult Services

The majority of adult service programs and agencies operate as eligibility services (Everson, 1993). In general, these services have specific criteria for entering and exiting the system. In contrast to special education, eligibility does not guarantee services, and the services are funded by multiple sources and operate within multiple agencies. Table 4.4 provides a summary of the major adult services and funding sources. Most of these services are funded as one of three types: employment services, social security and health care services, and community living and support services.

Employment Services

The major source of employment programs for adults with disabilities is the federal/state vocational rehabilitation (VR) program (Brown & Browning, 1997). Each state has a state rehabilitation system, funded through a combination of state and federal funds. Individuals interested in receiving VR services must meet the federally established eligibility criteria. Eligibility determination is made on a case-by-case basis. For a person to be eligible for VR services, the following must be established and documented: (a) the presence of a physical or mental disability that constitutes or results in a substantial handicap to employment and (b) a reasonable expectation that vocational rehabilitation services may benefit the individual in terms of employability (Rehabilitation Services Administration, 1976, § 1505.03). The kinds of services provided by VR programs include, but are not limited to, work evaluation, job counseling, job training, physical and mental restoration, financial assistance in education, interpreter services, and job placement and follow-up. Although the disability definitions for VR may differ from those of education agencies, determinations of disability from other agencies (e.g., local education agencies) can be used for the purpose of disability determination for VR (Brown & Browning, 1997).

With regard to transition, the 1992 Rehabilitation Act Reauthorization strengthened the language concerning interagency agreements, allowing for the establishment of interagency working groups and formal interagency cooperative agreements (National Transition Network, 1993b). Further, the act mandated that vocational rehabilitation agencies arrange for cooperation with the Social Security Administration and other federal and state agencies providing services to individuals with disabilities under IDEA, the Carl Perkins Act, and the Wagner-O'Day Act. Also, many state VR programs have rehabilitation counselors

(text continues on page 55)

TABLE 4.4
Summary of Major Adult Service Areas and Funding Sources

Employment Services	
Vocational Rehabilitation (VR) Program	Funds vocational evaluation, job training, and job placement services, as well as career counseling, medical and psychiatric services, and independent living services to eligible adults with disabilities. State agencies and local rehabilitation counselors may provide or purchase many of the specific employment services below. Authorized by the Rehabilitation Act, as amended.
Job Training Partnership Act (JTPA) Program	Funds disadvantaged youth, adult, displaced homemaker, Native American, migrant worker, and older American employment services. Federally funded by the U.S. Department of Labor and locally administered by private sector–organized Private Industry Councils (PICs). Authorized by the Job Training Partnership Act, as amended.
Transitional Employment Services	Time-limited, facility, or community-based employment for individuals with a range of disabilities. Provided as individual or group placements and includes the Project With Industry (PWI) model. Funded by state and federal rehabilitation funds and authorized by the Rehabilitation Act, as amended.
Supported Employment Services	Community-based employment with ongoing follow-along services for individuals with severe disabilities. Provided as individual or group placements known as job coach, supported work, supported jobs, enclaves, mobile work crews, or entrepreneurial models. Funded by state and federal rehabilitation and MR/DD funds and authorized by the Rehabilitation Act, as amended.
Sheltered Employment Services	Facility-based vocational preparation and employment for individuals with a range of disabilities. Facility obtains work contracts from major businesses and sheltered employees complete contracts within facility. Funded by state and federal rehabilitation and MR/DD funds and authorized by the Rehabilitation Act, as amended.
Day Activity/Day Treatment/Day Training Services	Facility-based rehabilitation or prevocational training for individuals with severe disabilities. Activities of daily living, leisure, and job readiness are typically provided. Funded by MR/DD funds.
Targeted Jobs Tax Credit (TJTC)	A special tax credit to induce businesses to hire employees with disabilities, disadvantaged youths, welfare recipients, and other hard-to-place workers. Authorized by The Tax Reform Act, as amended.
Social Security and Health Care Services	
Social Security Disability Insurance (SSDI)	Provides disability insurance in the form of monthly payments to disabled individuals with a work history who have paid into the Social Security system. Minor or disabled children of SSDI recipients are also eligible. Does not require a financial needs test. Funded and authorized by the Social Security Act, as amended.
Supplemental Security Income (SSI)	Provides monthly cash assistance to needy, aged and disabled individuals with little or no work history. Requires a financial needs test. Funded and authorized by the Social Security Act, as amended.

(continues)

TABLE 4.4 *Continued.*

Medicaid	Hospital and health care insurance for eligible poor and disabled persons. Federally regulated and state administered under the Social Security Act, as amended. Typically accompanies SSI benefits.
Medicare	Hospital and healthcare insurance for eligible elderly and disabled persons. Federally regulated and administered by the Social Security Act, as amended. Typically accompanies SSDI benefits.
Community Living and Support Services	
Intermediate Care Facilities for the Mentally Retarded (ICF-MR) Program	Medicaid-funded residences for children and adults with mental retardation or related conditions. Programs must conform to strict facility structure and client programming federal regulations. ICF-MR programs may be as large as public institutions or as small as 4- to 15-person group homes. Skilled nursing facilities (SNFs) and intermediate care facilities (ICFs) provide varying levels of nursing and medical services. Funded by Title XIX of the Social Security Acts, as amended.
Housing and Urban Development (HUD) Program	Federally administered and state authorized housing assistance program that provides low-cost loans (Section 202) to finance construction or rehabilitation of residential facilities for persons who are elderly or disabled. Section 202 may provide funding for the development of apartment complexes known as independent living complexes (ILCs) of up to 24 units per site and for group homes of up to 15 clients. Also provides rental aid (Section 8) to low-income families and individuals and to persons who are handicapped and not elderly (Section 162). Community Development Block Grants (CDBGs) are given to local communities by HUD to housing projects benefitting low- and moderate-income persons. They are generally in the form of below-market interest loans.
Group Homes/Supported Apartments	Community-based or institutional grounds–based residences of two or more individuals with disabilities and support staff. May or may not be regulated by ICF-MR funds. May or may not be accredited by the Accreditation Council for Facilities for the Developmentally Disabled (ACDD) or the Commission Accreditation of Rehabilitation Facilities (CARF). Typically provide structured community- and residence-based programming and require residents to attend a day program such as a sheltered workshop or a supported employment option. Also known as supported homes, community care homes, and community living alternatives (CLAs).
Adult Board and Care Homes	Community-based homes of various sizes that provide room and board for adults with disabilities. Typically, they provide minimal supervision and resident programming.
Food Stamps	Provides stamps that may be exchanged for food at grocery stores. Families, individuals, and groups of individuals (such as group home residents) are eligible depending on income and financial need. Typically, SSI recipients are eligible. Federally funded through the Department of Agriculture and state and locally administered by social service agencies.

Note. From *Youth with Disabilities: Strategies for Interagency Transition Programs* (pp. 8–9), by J. M. Everson, 1993, Austin, TX: PRO-ED. Copyright 1993 by PRO-ED, Inc. Reprinted with permission.

designated as "transition" counselors (Brown & Browning, 1997). These counselors work primarily with high school students, helping to prepare them for the transition from high school. Individuals can consult the phone directory or a school guidance counselor to locate the vocational rehabilitation office in their local community.

Social Security and Health Care Services

Another important funding source for adult services is Social Security, which directs two programs that can provide financial benefits to eligible individuals with disabilities throughout the transition process (Everson, 1993; NICHCY, 1991). The *Supplemental Security Income* (SSI) program is for individuals who are both in financial need and blind or disabled. Those who are eligible receive a monthly benefit check. Eligibility requirements vary depending upon the age of the individual. Those over the age of 18 are eligible to receive monthly payments if they (a) have little or no income or resources, (b) are medically disabled or blind, and (c) do not work or earn less than the amount established by the Social Security Administration as Substantial Gainful Activity (SGA). A change in employment status can result in a reduction or termination of benefits. Health care benefits for SSI recipients are provided through Medicaid.

The *Social Security Disability Insurance* (SSDI) program differs from SSI in that it considers the employment status of an individual's parents. SSDI is a disability insurance program that was initially established for workers who became disabled and were unable to return to work (Everson, 1993). Benefits are paid to individuals who become disabled before the age of 22 if one of their parents had worked a specified amount of time and then acquired a disability, retired, or died. Health care benefits for SSDI recipients are provided through Medicare programs.

Eligibility for SSI and SSDI usually makes an individual eligible for food stamps. Both programs are typically administered by the state's social services agency within federal Social Security Act regulations (Everson, 1993). In the past, income from a job would substantially reduce or even eliminate the amount of benefits. This was often seen as a disincentive for work. To address this concern, recent legislation has made major changes in these programs to encourage recipients to seek employment and become independent (NICHCY, 1991). SSI work incentives include allowing most individuals to keep Medicaid and state-funded attendant care benefits after they stop receiving monthly SSI checks and deducting impairment-related work expenses from earnings for the purpose of determining the SGA amount. SSI also provides for the development of a Plan for Achieving Self Support (PASS), which enables a person to receive earned and unearned income and to set aside some or all of the funds for the purpose of accumulating resources to be used to pursue a specific work goal (e.g., education, vocational training, starting a business). SSDI work incentives also include deducting work-related work expenses from earnings and extending Medicare coverage, as well as a trial work period.

Community Living and Support Services

A wide range of community living and support services are funded by a variety of federal, state, and local sources. The Intermediate Care Facilities for the Mentally Retarded (ICF-MR) program is one of the largest, funding residential care and related services for individuals with mental retardation and other related conditions who need 24-hour care. Such programs are usually administered by the state mental retardation or developmental disabilities agency within federal Social Security Act regulations. Because of opposition to the highly regimented nature of ICF-MR programs, smaller group homes, foster care, adult boarding homes, and supported apartments are more common in many states. These residential arrangements are usually funded and administered by the state and local agency of mental retardation or developmental disabilities using federal, state, and local dollars (Everson, 1993). Advocacy and parent groups are also involved in providing residential services as subcontractors or private corporations. Additionally, through the Developmental Disabilities Assistance and Bill of Rights Act, state-level Developmental Disabilities Planning Councils have been established to work with developmental disabilities state agencies for the purposes of developing a state plan for the provision of services.

TRANSITION TEAMS

As previously mentioned, education agencies historically have "owned" the transition movement because of their charge to serve individuals with disabilities through age 22 (Everson, 1993). Successful transition programs have realized, however, the essentialness of collaborating with rehabilitation and other adult service agencies in planning and service delivery. Further, addressing key transition issues requires "the resources of and expertise of several agencies and professional disciplines across federal, state, local, and individual student or client levels" (Everson, 1993, p. 11). Consequently, interagency transition teams have been established at several levels to address key transition issues.

Blalock (1996) identified five levels of transition teams. At the individual student level, there is an *individualized transition planning* (ITP) committee. This team's focus is on the development and implementation of transition plans for individual students. This team meets at least annually for each student, to evaluate progress toward and reevaluate the appropriateness of long-term goals. At the school level, *school-based transition committees* address general issues affecting transition programming. For example, curricular changes, the development of transition planning procedures, and the integration of vocational assessment into transition planning are issues that could be addressed by a school-based team. Blalock (1996) noted that existing school-based teams, such as building-based curriculum committees and student support teams, could serve in such a capacity or a team might evolve to specifically address transition education. *Community and regional transition teams* address a broader range of issues, focusing on improved secondary and adult services, programs, and life choices. Because the purpose of community and regional teams is similar, typically a state would have only one of the levels (Blalock, 1996). These teams assess, plan, change, monitor, and evaluate transition efforts within the community or region. Issues addressed by such teams could include improving interagency collaboration, creating community training and employment opportunities, and addressing transportation and housing issues. Finally, at the state level, *state-level transition teams* consider state policy and regulations relating to transition. Blalock (1996) noted that the efforts at this level are directed primarily toward opening the doors for interagency collaboration at the state level, with the intent of enhancing collaboration at the local level.

Although the benefits and accomplishments of all levels of transition teams are numerous and the initiative for increasing interagency collaboration has been established at the federal level through joint policy statements between various agencies, including special education, community health services, vocational education, and vocational rehabilitation, the reality is that implementation of cooperative efforts at the state, regional or community, school, and even individual level is often problematic (Johnson, Bruininks, & Thurlow, 1987). Numerous challenges face teams at all levels. Johnson et al. (1987) suggested that conflicting policy goals, eligibility criteria, funding patterns, and other variables that differ across agencies make it difficult to provide and coordinate appropriate services. Edgar, Horton, and Maddox (1984) noted that (a) inconsistent organizational patterns across agencies, (b) discontinuity in the geographic areas covered by programs, (c) differing application procedures for eligibility, and (d) varying planning cycles and fiscal years often interfere with the successful transition of persons with developmental disabilities from the public schools to appropriate community services.

CHAPTER 5
Epilogue

The transition planning process requires that certain key elements—assessment, individual planning, follow-through, and coordination (see Figure 1.2)—be executed in a timely fashion. As mentioned in Chapter 1 and depicted in Figure 1.3, this is a shared process, involving school-based personnel, the student, the family, and a variety of adult service providers. As a concluding thought for this book, it is useful to highlight important ways that these four key entities can best contribute to this planning process. The following lists represent an evolution of thinking that was originally begun by a group of professionals connected to the Hawaii Transition Project (1987).

How Schools Can Best Prepare Students for Adulthood

- Address proactively the important life skills within the curriculum.
- Develop self-determination/self-advocacy skills in students.
- Assess and plan comprehensively for transitional needs.
- Provide community-based experiences.
- Assist families in dealing with the adult service arena.

How Families Can Ensure Successful Transition

- Become informed about the demands of adulthood and the transition planning process.
- Participate actively in the transition process.
- Follow through on designated linkage activities.
- Seek assistance when needed.
- Advocate for their children.

How Students Can Contribute to the Transition Effort

- Identify their own preferences and interests.
- Take an interest in this process.
- Participate as a contributing member of their transition team.
- Follow through on designated activities.
- Know where and how to access supports and services.

How Adult Service Providers Can Facilitate Successful Transition

- Identify the demands and requisite skills needed in their particular settings or programs.
- Provide information about their settings or programs to school-based personnel.
- Participate in the transition process when feasible.
- Offer accessibility and assistance to families.

It is unlikely that the type of transition planning process that we keep discussing will ever be in place. However, armed with the knowledge of what could be and motivated by what is important for those students who are leaving school and venturing out into the community, transition professionals have the opportunity to make a difference in the lives of many young adults. All that we, as professionals, do must be guided by a desire to provide these young adults with the knowledge, skills, supports, and services that will enhance their lives and, in some way, contribute to their experiencing some degree of personal fulfillment.

Jerry Seinfeld, in his book *SeinLanguage* (1993), may have captured the essence of our mission as educators in preparing students for the challenges of adulthood:

> Life is truly a ride. We're all strapped in and no one can stop it. When the doctor slaps your behind, he's ripping your ticket and away you go. As you make each passage from youth to adulthood to maturity, sometimes you put your arms up and scream, sometimes you just hang on to that bar in front of you. But the ride is the thing. I think the most you can hope for at the end of life is that your hair's messed, you're out of breath, and you didn't throw up. (p. 153)

Here's to the ride and those who prepare students for it.

Appendix

National Organizations and Resources

Alexander Graham Bell Association for the Deaf
3417 Volta Place NW
Washington, DC 20007
202/337-5220 (voice & TTY)
www.agbell.org

American Association of Community Colleges
One Dupont Circle NW
Suite 410
Washington, DC 20036
202/728-0200

American Association on Mental Retardation
444 North Capitol Street NW
Washington DC 20001-1512
800/424-3688
www.aamr.org

American Camping Association
Project on Science, Technology and Disability
1333 H Street NW
Washington, DC 20005
410/484-1409
www.camps.org

American Council of the Blind
1155 15th Street NW
Suite 720
Washington, DC 20005
800/424-8666
www.acb.org

American Society for the Deaf
814 Thayer Avenue
Silver Springs, MD 20852
301/585-5400

American Foundation for the Blind
11 Penn Plaza
Suite 300
New York, NY 10001
212/620-2000

American Vocational Association
1410 King Street
Alexandria, VA 22314
800/826-9972

American Wheelchair Bowling Association
N54 W15858 Larkspur Lane
Menomonee Falls, WI 53051
414/781-6876

The Arc
500 East Border Street
Suite 300
Arlington, TX 76010
817/261-6003
www.thearc.org

Association for Education of the Visually Handicapped
919 Walnut Street
4th Floor
Philadelphia, PA 19107

Association for Persons in Supported Employment
5001 West Broad Street
Suite 34
Richmond, VA 23230
804/282-3655

Association on Higher Education and Disability (AHEAD)
P.O. Box 21192
Columbus, OH 43221
614/488-4972

Beach Center on Families and Disability
Bureau of Child Research
University of Kansas
3111 Haworth Hall
Lawrence, KS 66045
913/864-7600
www.lsi.ukans.edu/beach/beachhp.htm

Breckenridge Outdoor Education Center
P.O. Box 697
Breckenridge, CO 80424
970/453-6422
www.brecknet.com/bocc

Children and Adults with Attention Deficit Disorder (CHADD)
499 Northwest 70th Avenue
Suite 308
Plantation, FL 33317
305/587-3700
www.chadd.org

Clearinghouse on Disability Information
Office of Special Education and Rehabilitative Services
U.S. Department of Education, Room 3132
Switzer Building
Washington, DC 20202-2542
202/732-1723

Connecticut Post Secondary Disability Technical Assistance Center
The University of Connecticut, U-64
249 Glenbrook Road
Storrs, CT 06269-2064
860/486-0273
www.ucc.uconn.edu/~wwwpcse/pedu.htm

Closer Look LD Teen Line
1201 16th Street
Suite 223
Washington, DC 20036
800/522-3458

The Council of Exceptional Children
1920 Association Drive
Reston, VA 22091
703/620-3660
www.cec.step.org

Disabled and Alone/Life Services for the Handicapped, Inc.
352 Park Avenue South
Suite 703
New York, NY 10010
800/995-0066

Division of Adult Education and Literacy Clearinghouse
U.S. Department of Education
Office of Vocational and Adult Education
400 Maryland Avenue SW
Washington, DC 20202
202/205-9996

Division of Career Development and Transition
Council for Exceptional Children
1920 Association Drive
Reston, VA 22091-1589
703/620-3660

Dole Foundation for the Employment of Persons with Disabilities
1819 H Street NW
Suite 340
Washington, DC 20006
202/457-0318

Education Resources Information Center (ERIC)
National Clearinghouse on Literacy Education
Center for Applied Linguistics
Washington, DC 20013
202/429-9292

ERIC Clearinghouse on Adult, Career, and Vocational Counseling
Ohio State University
Center on Education and Training for Employment
1900 Kenny Road
Columbus, OH 43210-1090
800/848-4815

Gallaudet University
800 Florida Avenue NE
Washington, DC 20002
202/651-5000

HEATH Resource Center
One Dupont Circle
Suite 800
Washington, DC 20036-1193
800/544-3284

Helen Keller National Center–Technical Assistance Center (TAC)
111 Middle Neck Road
Sands Point, NY 11050-1299
516/944-8900

Independent Living Research Utilization Program
2323 South Shepherd
Suite 1000
Houston, TX 77019
713/520-0232

Institute on Community Integration
University of Minnesota
109 Pattee Hall
150 Pillsbury Drive SE
Minneapolis, MN 55455

Job Accommodation Network (JAN)
918 Chestnut Ridge Road
P.O. Box 6080
Morgantown, WV 26506
800/526-7234
www.janweb.icdi.wvu.edu

Job Opportunities for the Blind (JOB)
National Federation of the Blind
1800 Johnson Street
Baltimore, MD 21230
800/683-7518

Jobs for the Future
Student Apprenticeship News
Cambridge, MA
617/661-4311

Laubach Literacy Action (LLA)
P.O. Box 131
Syracuse, NY 13210
315/422-9121

Learning Disabilities Association of America
4156 Library Road
Pittsburg, PA 15234
412/341-1515
www.ldanatl.org

Life Development Institute
P.O. Box 15112
Phoenix, AZ 85060
602/955-2920

Life Services for the Handicapped, Inc.
352 Park Avenue South
New York, NY 10010

Literacy Volunteers of America (LVA)
5795 Widewaters Parkway
Syracuse, NY 13214
315/335-8000

Material Development Center (MDC)
Stout Vocational Rehabilitation Institute
University of Wisconsin at Stout
Menomonee, WI 54751
715/232-1342

National Association for Visually Handicapped (NAVH)
22 West 21st Street
New York, NY 10010
212/889-3141
www.navh.org

National Association of Private Residential Facilities for the Mentally Retarded
6269 Leesburg Pike, Suite B5
Falls Church, VA 22044

National Association of Vocational Education Special Needs Personnel (NAVESNP)
Special Needs Division
American Vocational Association
2020 14th Street
Arlington, VA 22201
703/522-6121

National Center for Research in Vocational Education
2150 Shattuck Avenue
Suite 1250
Berkeley, CA 24704
800/762-4093

National Center on Disability Services
201 I.U. Willets Road
Albertson, NY 11507

National Center on Independent Living
310 South Peoria Street
Suite 201
Chicago, IL 60607

National Clearinghouse on Postsecondary Education for Individuals with Disabilities (HEATH Resource Center)
One Dupont Circle
Suite 800
Washington, DC 20036-1193
800/544-3284

National Clearinghouse on Women and Girls with Disabilities
Educational Equities Concepts, Inc.
114 East 32nd Street
Suite 701
New York, NY 10016
212/725-1803
www.onisland.com/eec.wwd

National Council for Youth with Disabilities/Institute Health & Disability
University of Minnesota
Box 721, 420 Delaware Street SE
Minneapolis, MN 55455
612/626-2825
www.peds.umn.edu/centers/ncyd

National Council of Independent Living Programs (NCIL)
2111 Wilson Boulevard
Suite 40
Arlington, VA 22201
703/525-3406

National Council on Independent Living
2111 Wilson Boulevard
Suite 405
Arlington, VA 22201
703/525-3406

National Down's Syndrome Congress (NDSC)
1640 West Roosevelt Road
Chicago, IL 60608
800/232-6372

National Handicapped Sports
4405 East-West Highway # 603
Bethesda, MD 20814

National Industries for the Blind
524 Hamburg Turnpike
CN969
Wayne, NJ 07474-0969
201/595-9200

National Industries for the Severely Handicapped
2235 Cedar Lane
Vienna, VA 22180
703/560-6800

National Information Center for Children and Youth with Disabilities (NICHCY)
P.O. Box 1492
Washington, DC 20013
800/695-0285
www.nichcy.org

National Information Center on Deafness
Gallaudet University
800 Florida Avenue, NE
Washington, DC 20002
202/651-5051
www.gallaudet.edu/~nicd

National Parent Network on Disabilities
1600 Prince Street
Suite 115
Alexandria, VA 22314

National Rehabilitation Information Center (NARIC)
8455 Colesville Road
Suite 935
Silver Spring, MD 20910
800/322-0956
www.naric.com/naric

National Tech Prep Network
Center for Occupational Research and Development
P.O. Box 21689
Waco, TX 76702-1689
800/972-2766

National Transition Network
Institute on Community Integration
University of Minnesota
Pattee Hall
150 Pillsbury Drive SE
Minneapolis, MN 55455

Office of Vocational and Adult Education
U.S. Department of Education
Washington, DC
202/205-5440

Office of Work-Based Learning
U.S. Department of Labor
Washington, DC
202/219-5281

PACER Center, Inc.
4826 Chicago Avenue South
Minneapolis, MN 55417-1098
800/53-PACER
www.pacer.org

Parents Advocating Vocational Education (PAVE)
6316 South 12th Street
Tacoma, WA 98465
800/572-7368

President's Committee on Employment of Persons with Disabilities (PCEPD)
1331 F Street NW
Washington, DC 20004
202/376-6200

Recording for the Blind and Dyslexic
20 Roszel Road
Princeton, NJ 20542
800/221-4792
www.rfbd.org

The Research and Training Center on Independent Living
University of Kansas
4089 Dole Building
Lawrence, KS 66045
913/864-4095 (voice/TT)
www.lsi.ukans.edu/rtcil/rtcbroc.htm

Secondary Transition Intervention Institute
Transition Institute at Illinois
University of Illinois
College of Education
110 Education Building
1310 South 6th Street
Champaign, IL 61820
217/333-2325

Shared Outdoor Adventure Recreation (SOAR)
P.O. Box 14583
Portland, OR 14583

Social Security Administration
U.S. Department of Health and Human Services
1801 L Street NW
Washington, DC 20507
800/772-1213

Technical Assistance for Parent Program (TAPP)
Federation of Children with Special Needs
95 Berkeley Street
Boston, MA 02116
800/331-0688

Technical Assistance for Special Population Program (TASPP)
National Center for Research in Vocational Education (NCRVE)
University of Illinois
345 Education Building
1310 South 6th Street
Champaign, IL 61820

Virginia Commonwealth University Rehabilitation Research and Training Center on Supported Employment (RRTC)
RRTC
Virginia Commonwealth University
1314 West Main Street
Richmond, VA 23284-2011

Postsecondary Guides

Branson, J. P. (1987). *A guide to higher education for learning disabled students.* Coatesville, PA: Chester County Intermediate Unit. (Available from Chester County Intermediate Unit, 1530 East Lincoln Highway, Coatesville, PA 19320)

Fielding, P. M., & Fabian-Isaacs, C. (Eds.). (1993). *National directory of four year colleges, two year colleges and post high school training programs for young people with learning disabilities.* Tulsa, OK: Partners in Publishing. (Available from Partners in Publishing, Box 50347, Tulsa, OK 74150)

Kravetz, M., & Wax, I. F. (1996). *The K&W guide to colleges for the learning disabled: A resource book for students, parents, and professionals* (4th ed.). Princeton, NJ: Princeton Review. (Available from Random House, 400 Hahn Road, Westminster, MD 21157)

Lipkin, M. (1990). *Guide to college programs or services for students with learning disabilities.* Belmont, MA: Schoolsearch Press. (Available from Schoolsearch Press, 127 March Street, Belmont, MA 02178)

Rawlings, B., Karchmer, M., & DeCaro, J. J. (Eds.). (1991). *College and career programs for deaf students.* Washington, DC: Gallaudet College and National Technical Institute for the Deaf. (Available from Office of Demographic Studies, Gallaudet College, 800 Florida Avenue NE, Washington, DC 20002-3625)

Skyer, R., & Skyer, G. (1986). *What do you do after high school? A nationwide guide to residential, vocational, social, and collegiate programs serving the adolescent, young adult, and adult with learning disabilities.* Rockaway Park, NY: Skyer Consultation Center, Inc. (Available from Skyer Consultation Center, Inc., P.O. Box 121, Rockaway Park, NY 11694)

Slovak, I. (Ed.). (1990). *BOSC directory for facilities for learning disabled.* Congers, NY: BOSC. (Available from BOSC, Dept. F, Box 305, Congers, NY 10920)

Straughn, C. T. (1993). *Lovejoy's college guide for the learning disabled.* New York: Monarch Press. (Available from Macmillan, 1230 Avenue of the Americas, New York, NY 10020)

Tweed, P. K., & Tweed, J. C. (1989). *Colleges that enable: A guide to support services offered to physically disabled students on 40 U.S. campuses.* New Wilmington, PA: Park Avenue Press. (Available from Jason Tweed, 4B Tanglewood Drive, Reading, PA 19607)

References

Armstrong, D. G. (1989). *Developing and documenting the curriculum.* Boston: Allyn & Bacon.

Beirne-Smith, M., Ittenbach, R., & Patton, J. (1998). *Mental retardation* (5th ed.). New York: Prentice-Hall/Merrill Education.

Bennett, G. K., Seashore, H. G., & Wesman, A. G. (1990). *Differential Aptitude Tests, Fifth Edition.* San Antonio: Harcourt Brace Educational Measurement.

Blalock, G. (1996). Community transition teams as the foundation for transition services for youth with learning disabilities. *Journal of Learning Disabilities, 29,* 148–159.

Blalock, G., & Patton, J. R. (1996). Transition and students with learning disabilities: Creating sound futures. *Journal of Learning Disabilities, 29,* 7–16.

Brigance, A. H. (1995). *Life Skills Inventory.* North Billerica, MA: Curriculum Associates.

Brolin, D. E. (1992). *Life-Centered Career Education (LCCE) Knowledge and Performance Batteries.* Reston, VA: Council for Exceptional Children.

Brolin, D. E. (1993). *Life centered career education: A competency-based approach* (4th ed.). Reston, VA: The Council for Exceptional Children.

Brown, C., & Browning, P. (1997). School to work linked practices. In P. Browning (Ed.), *Transition in action for youth and young adults with disabilities* (pp. 207–240). Montgomery, AL: Wells Printing.

Brown, L., Shiraga, B., York, J., Kessler, K., Strohm, B., Rogan, P., Sweet, M., Zanella, K., VanDeventer, P., & Loomis, R. (1984). Integrated work opportunities for adults with severe handicaps: The extended training options. *The Journal of the Association for Persons with Severe Handicaps, 9,* 262–269.

Clark, G. M. (1996). Transition planning assessment for secondary-level students with learning disabilities. *Journal of Learning Disabilities, 29,* 79–92.

Clark, G. M. (1998). *Assessment for transition planning.* Austin, TX: PRO-ED.

Clark, G. M., Carlson, B. C., Fisher, S., Cook, I. D., & D'Alonzo, B. J. (1991). Career development for students with disabilities in elementary schools: A position statement of the Division on Career Development. *Career Development for Exceptional Individuals, 14,* 109–120.

Clark, G. M., Field, S., Patton, J. R., Brolin, D. E., & Sitlington, P. L. (1994). Life skills instruction: A necessary component for all students with disabilities. A position statement of the Division on Career Development and Transition. *Career Development for Exceptional Individuals, 17,* 125–134.

Clark, G. M., & Kolstoe, O. P. (1995). *Career development and transition education for adolescents with disabilities* (2nd ed.). Boston: Allyn & Bacon.

Clark, G. M., & Patton, J. R. (1997). *Transition Planning Inventory.* Austin, TX: PRO-ED.

Clees, T. (1992). Community living. In P. J. McLaughlin & P. Wehman (Eds.), *Developmental disabilities: A handbook for best practices* (pp. 228–267). Boston: Andover Medical.

Condeluci, A. (1995). *Interdependence: The route to community* (2nd ed.). Winter Park, FL: GR Press.

Crawford, J. (1981). *Crawford Small Parts Dexterity Test.* San Antonio: Psychological Corp.

Cronin, M. E., & Patton, J. R. (1993). *Life skills instruction for all students with special needs: A practical guide for integrating real-life content into the curriculum.* Austin, TX: PRO-ED.

deFur, S., & Patton, J. R. (Eds.). (in press). *Transition and school-based services: Interdisciplinary perspectives for enhancing the transition process.* Austin, TX: PRO-ED.

deFur, S., & Reiff, H. B. (1994). Transition of youths with learning disabilities to adulthood: The secondary education foundation. In P. J. Gerber & H. B. Reiff (Eds.), *Learning disabilities in adulthood: Persisting problems and evolving issues* (p. 99–110). Austin, TX: PRO-ED.

Dever, R. B. (1988). *Community living skills: A taxonomy.* Washington, DC: American Association on Mental Retardation.

Dowdy, C., & Evers, R. (1996). Preparing students for transition: A teacher primer on vocational education and rehabilitation. *Intervention in School and Clinic, 31,* 197–208.

Dunn, C., & Rabren, K. (1997). Preparation practices. In P. Browning (Ed.), *Transition in action for youth and young adults with disabilities* (pp. 173–204). Montgomery, AL: Wells Printing.

Dunn, R., Dunn, K., & Price, G. E. (1995). *Learning Styles Inventory.* Lawrence, KS: Price Systems.

Edgar, E., Horton, B., & Maddox, M. (1984). Postschool placements: Planning for public school students with developmental disabilities. *The Journal of Vocational Special Needs, 6*(2), 15–18, 26.

Education for All Handicapped Children Act of 1975, 20 U.S.C. § 1400 *et seq.*

Enderle, J., & Severson, S. (1997). *Enderle–Severson Transition Rating Scale–Revised.* Moorehead, MN: Practical Press.

Everson, J. M. (1993). *Youth with disabilities: Strategies for interagency transition programs.* Austin, TX: PRO-ED.

Gajar, A., Goodman, L., & McAfee, J. (1993). *Secondary schools and beyond: Transition of individuals with mild disabilities.* New York: Merrill.

Halpern, A. S. (1985). Transition: A look at the foundations. *Exceptional Children, 51,* 479–486.

Halpern, A. S. (1993). Quality of life as a conceptual framework for evaluating transition outcomes. *Exceptional Children, 59,* 486–498.

Halpern, A. S. (1994). The transition of youth with disabilities to adult life: A position statement of the Division on Career Development and Transition, The Council for Exceptional Children. *Career Development for Exceptional Individuals, 17,* 115–124.

Halpern, A. S., & Benz, M. R. (1987). A statewide examination of secondary special education for students with mild disabilities: Implications for the high school curriculum. *Exceptional Children, 54,* 122–129.

Halpern, A. S., Herr, C. M., Wolf, N. K., Doren, B., Johnson, M. D., & Lawson, J. D. (1997). *Next S.T.E.P.: Student transition and educational planning.* Austin, TX: PRO-ED.

Halpern, A. S., Irvin, L., & Landman, J. J. (1979). *Tests for Everyday Living.* Monterey, CA: CTB/McGraw-Hill.

Halpern, A. S., Irvin, L., & Munkres, J. (1986). *Social and Prevocational Information Battery–Revised.* Monterey, CA: CTB/McGraw-Hill.

Hasazi, S. B., Gordon, L. B., & Roe, C. A. (1985). Factors associated with the employment status of handicapped youth exiting from high school from 1979 to 1983. *Exceptional Children, 51,* 455–469.

Hawaii Transition Project. (1987). Honolulu: University of Hawaii, Department of Special Education.

Helmke, L. M., Havekost, D. M., Patton, J. R., & Polloway, E. A. (1994). Life skills programming: Development of a high school science course. *Teaching Exceptional Children, 26*(2), 49–53.

Heward, W. (1996). *Exceptional children: An introduction to special education* (5th ed.). Columbus, OH: Merrill.

Holland, A. L. (1980). *Communicative Abilities in Daily Living.* Austin, TX: PRO-ED.

Jackson, D. N. (1995). *Basic Personality Inventory.* Port Huron, MI: Sigma Assessment Systems.

Johnson, D. R., Bruininks, R. H., & Thurlow, M. L. (1987). Meeting the challenge of transition service planning through improved interagency cooperation. *Exceptional Children, 53,* 522–530.

Jones, M., & Ulciny, G. (1986). The independent living perspective: Application to services for adults with developmental living. In J. Summers (Ed.), *The right to group up: An introduction to adults with developmental disabilities* (pp. 227–244). Baltimore: Brookes.

Karlsen, B., & Gardner, E. (1986). *Adult Basic Learning Examination–Second Edition.* San Antonio: Harcourt Brace Educational Measurement.

Keith, K. D., & Schalock, R. L. (1995). *Quality of Student Life Questionnaire.* Worthington, OH: IDS.

Klein, J. (1994). Supported living: Not just another "rung" on the continuum. *TASH Newsletter, 20*(7) 16–18.

Knowles, M. (1990). *The adult learner: The neglected species.* Houston: Gulf.

Lambert, N., Nihira, K., & Leland, H. (1993). *AAMR Adaptive Behavior Scales–School: Second Edition.* Austin, TX: PRO-ED.

Luckasson, R., Coulter, D. L., Polloway, E. A., Reiss, S., Shalock, R. L., Snell, M. E., Spitalnik, D. M., & Stark, J. A. (1992). *Mental retardation: Definition, classification, and systems of supports* (9th ed.). Washington, DC: American Association on Mental Retardation.

Martin, J. E., Huber Marshall, L. H., Maxson, L., & Jerman, P. (1996). *Self-directed IEP.* Longmont, CO: Sopris West.

McCarney, S. B. (1989). *Transition Behavior Scale.* Columbia, MO: Hawthorne Educational Service.

Minskoff, E. (1994). Post-secondary education and vocational training: Keys to success for adults with learning disabilities. In P. Gerber & H. Reiff (Eds.), *Learning disabilities in adulthood: Persisting problems and evolving issues* (pp. 111–120). Boston: Andover Medical.

Mithaug, D. E., Horiuchi, C. N., & Fanning, P. N. (1985). A report on the Colorado statewide follow-up survey of special education students. *Exceptional Children, 51,* 397–404.

National Association of Secondary School Principals. (1996). *Breaking ranks: Changing an American institution.* Reston, VA: Author.

National Center on Educational Outcomes. (1993). *Education outcomes and indicators for individuals at the post-school level.* Minneapolis: University of Minnesota.

National Information Center for Children and Youth with Disabilities. (1991, September). *Options after high school for youth with disabilities* (Transition Summary, No. 7). Washington, DC: Author.

National Transition Network. (1993a, Winter). IDEA: Its impact on transition regulations. *Policy Update,* pp. 1–4. Minneapolis: University of Minnesota, Institute on Community Integration.

National Transition Network. (1993b, Spring). 1992 Rehabilitation Act Amendments: New requirements for transition. *Policy Update.* Minneapolis: University of Minnesota, Institute on Community Integration.

Parker, R. (1991). *Occupational Aptitude Survey and Interest Schedule* (2nd ed.). Austin, TX: PRO-ED.

Patton, J. R., Cronin, M. E., & Jairrels, V. (1997). Curricular implications of transition: Life skills instruction as an integral part of transition education. *Remedial and Special Education, 18,* 294–306.

Rehabilitation Services Administration. (1976). *Rehabilitation services manual.* Washington, DC: U.S. Department of Education, Office of Special Education and Rehabilitative Services, Rehabilitation Services Administration.

Schalock, R. L., & Keith, K. D. (1993). *Quality of Life Questionnaire.* Worthington, OH: IDS.

Scheiber, B., & Talpers, J. (1987). *Unlocking potential: College and other choices for learning disabled people. A step-by-step guide.* Bethesda, MD: Adler & Adler.

Schleien, S., Rynders, J., & Green, F. (1994). Facilitating integration in recreation environments. In M. Hayden & B. Abery (Eds.), *Challenges for a service system in transition: Ensuring quality community experiences for persons with developmental disabilities* (pp. 121–145). Baltimore: Brookes.

Schutz, R. P. (1988). New directions and strategies in habilitation services: Toward meaningful employment outcomes. In L. W. Heal, J. I. Haney, & A. R. Novak Amoado (Eds.), *Integration of developmentally disabled individuals into the community* (2nd ed., pp. 193–209). Baltimore: Brookes.

Seinfeld, J. (1993). *SeinLanguage.* New York: Bantam.

Sitlington, P. L. (1996). Transition to living: The neglected components of transition programming for individuals with learning disabilities. *Journal of Learning Disabilities, 29,* 31–39, 52.

Sitlington, P., Frank, A., & Carson, R. (1993). Adult adjustment among graduates with mild disabilities. *Exceptional Children, 59,* 221–233.

Sitlington, P. L., Neubert, D. A., Begun, W., Lombard, R. C., & Leconte, P. J. (1996). *Assess for success: Handbook on transition assessment.* Reston, VA: Division on Career Development and Transition, Council for Exceptional Children.

Smith, M. A., & Schloss, P. J. (1988). Teaching to transition. In P. J. Schloss, C. A. Hughes, & M. A. Smith (Eds.), *Community integration for persons with mental retardation* (pp. 1–16). Austin, TX: PRO-ED.

U. S. Department of Education. (1995). *17th annual report to Congress on the implementation of IDEA.* Washington, DC: Author.

Vogelsberg, R. T., & Schutz, R. P. (1988). Establishing community employment programs for persons with severe disabilities: Systems designs and resolutions. In M. D. Powers (Ed.), *Expanding systems of service delivery for persons with developmental disabilities* (pp. 127–147), Baltimore: Brookes.

Wagner, M., Blackorby, J., Cameto, R., Hebbeler, K., & Newman, L. (1993). *The transition experiences of young people with disabilities: A summary of findings from the National Longitudinal Transition Study of special education students.* Menlo Park, CA: SRI International.

Wagner, M., Newman, L., D'Amico, R., Jay, E. D., Butler-Nalin, P., Marder, C., & Cox, R. (1991). *Youth with disabilities: How are they doing? The first comprehensive report from the National Longitudinal Transition Study of special education students.* Menlo Park, CA: SRI International.

Wehman, P. (1979). *Recreation programming for developmentally disabled persons.* Baltimore: University Park Press.

Wehman, P. (1988). *Transition from school to work: New challenges for youth with severe disabilities.* Baltimore: Brookes.

Wehman, P. (1995). *Individual transition plans: The teacher's curriculum guide for helping youth with special needs.* Austin, TX: PRO-ED.

Wehman, P. (Ed.). (1998). *Developing transition plans.* Austin, TX: PRO-ED.

Will, M. (1984). *OSERS programming for the transition of youth with disabilities: Bridges from school to working life.* Washington, DC: Office of Special Education and Rehabilitative Services.